The Art of Birth

The Art of Birth

Empower Yourself

For Conception, Pregnancy and Birth

Alexandra Florschutz

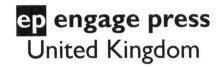 engage press
United Kingdom

First Published by engage press in 2013

The Art of Birth – Empower Yourself
For Conception, Pregnancy and Birth
Alexandra Florschutz

Cover Design: Lee Hannam at Yellowfishdesign
Interior Design: Ingrid Vienings

Published in the United Kingdom by engage press
ISBN: 978-0-9926555-1-8

Version 1
Printed by Lightning Source UK, a DBA of On-Demand Publishing, LLC

To my son Jude, my greatest teacher,
inspiration, joy and love.
This book would not exist without you.

Table of Contents

List of Art Images by Alexandra Florschutz

Disclaimer:

Every care has been taken to offer information that is correct, to the best of my knowledge, at the time of writing this book. All art exercises are tried and tested and although these can enable deeper personal insight, they do not guarantee a specific birth outcome. This book is intended for self development and to invite you to see birth as a defining event in your life. It is important to remember that whatever birth intervention you may have already experienced or might be necessary in the future, a healthy baby and mother is paramount. If at any point while reading this book or following the exercises and doing the inner work you feel the need for more support with emotions or issues that may arise, then please consult your doctor; find a suitable therapist/counsellor/art therapist; or you can contact me at alex@theartofbirth.co.uk and I can offer Skype™ sessions or email support.

I use the word 'her' and 'she' throughout the book when I talk about your baby. I find it preferable to using 'it', 'his/her' or 's/he and it includes the masculine.

Affirmations

The Archetypal Affirmations that run through this book have been created by Binnie A. Dansby, the founder of SOURCE Process and Breathwork Therapy, a unique approach to mind, body, spirit development. 'Thoughts to Remember' are also courtesy of Binnie.

Acknowledgements

To my son Jude who inspired me to write this book and who has been my greatest teacher, my true love and my hardest task master. I love you more than you could ever know and I thank you for the gift you have given me, to be your mother. To Bagus, Jude's father, thank you for loving me enough to marry me and co-create our son. My deepest thanks to my parents Gerhard and Liz Florschutz for their continued and unconditional love and support you have given to both Jude and me. Thank you. To Bella, my sister, thank you for always being there for me in so many ways and supporting my journey. I love you.

I want to thank Martin Keefe, David Thomas, Nick Tuckley and Jon Brody for your friendship, for supporting my physical wellbeing through massage, chiropractic treatments, osteopathy and acupuncture. This book would not have happened without your generosity. My heartfelt thanks to my dear friends and mentors, Binnie A. Dansby, Pat Bennaceur, Karel Ironside, Andy Beckingham (a.k.a. Beck) and Barry Durdant-Hollamby for your friendship and psychological support. I value your insightful teachings and wisdom which have all been an integral part of my journey. Jon Brody, Keith Weir and Seb Mower thank you for your unconditional technical support and design in looking after my faithful computer that wrote this book. And thank you computer. To all my friends who have contributed to the editing process: Emma Hiwaizi, Patricia Patterson-Vanegas, Jim Patterson, Martin, Isabella, Beck and Binnie thank you for taking your time to read the book and offer your comments. Thank you Ingrid Vienings for setting out the book so well and Lee Hannam of Yellowfishdesign for the beautiful book cover design.

And last but certainly not least all my dear friends who have helped me or stood by me over the years while I persevered studying, painting, writing this book and creating all my art. Thank you David Harbottle for your practical help and parenting support; to Seb Mower for website help; John Sleeman for publishing advice; to Alethea Mifsud for your unwavering support and friendship; Jacqui Grace for your friendship, your support in those challenging moments and for keeping me alight with fun, thank you. Christianne Key for your friendship and support, especially in those childcare moments, but also for keeping me motivated through lively discussion, guidance and laughter. To Patrick Houser, Nigel Grace, Sue Ashby, Sally Sampson, Lisette Wilson, and to all my other friends who help make my life as amazing as it is, thank you.

The Truth about Birth

Introduction

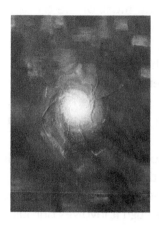

✦ **Birth can be an ecstatic experience for a woman – a rite of passage**

Every Human Being starts Life inside a Woman's body and yet Birth is feared by most Women – and Men. This is not surprising as over 50% of Births in the UK require medical intervention and this statistic is rising. Many of these Births can be traumatic for the Mother, not to mention the Baby. Birth is our entrance into this world and it has an impact that stays with us throughout life. If we can heal the fears, emotional barriers and life diminishing thought patterns that hinder the natural, pleasurable flow of Birth, then we can birth our babies – the future generations of this planet – more peacefully. We can do this by exploring our inner world using Expressive Art to gain deeper clarity and help us create the pregnancy and birth we desire. I have discovered that art and birth are compatible because they are both creative processes that harness our vital life energy. Art is physical, spiritual, intuitive and tangible and offers a valuable way back to our authentic Selves. Through carefully designed art exercises, affirmations, relaxation meditations and pleasure, you will have the tools to navigate your internal landscape and connect to your inherent wisdom. Let us reclaim birth as a rite of passage for Women (and Men) as powerful givers of life. Let us, once again, take Birth into our own hands. My personal story, the catalyst for my positive birth experience and general life change, underpins the book. I also include my art work which charts my creative journey, a parallel journey from conception to motherhood. This exciting and unique book, promises to be not only informative but very much 'transformative' for anyone who is interested in being a conscious person. We are all connected and so we all share the responsibility for supporting a positive outcome for new life and thus creating an overall paradigm shift for birth. If we approach birth in a conscious, positive, loving and gentle way, then we have the opportunity to manifest this shift.

⊥ Well begun is half done (Maharishi)

Women have all the physical and most of the emotional responsibility for birth, an enormous life-changing task, and yet they receive very little support or validation for this role. We are collectively accountable for ensuring pregnancy and birth is a positive experience for mother and baby and, of course, for the father. It is assumed nowadays that women just 'give birth' and yet most births could be much more pleasurable. In the west, birth is seen as painful, potentially traumatic or even dangerous and, at times, these assumptions become a self-fulfilling prophesy.

The Art of Birth invites you to consider the possibility that pregnancy, birth and parenting CAN happen in gentle and conscious ways that can change the world for future generations. Birth is potentially the most sacred, positive and wonderful experience in the world, even though it involves our full participation, energy and focus.

Through my research and my story I describe how it may be possible to move cultural consciousness about birth, from a fear-based paradigm to one of empowerment linked with a mother's inner world. *The Art of Birth* aims to inspire, educate and support pregnant women, midwives, doulas, childbirth practitioners, fathers, women/couples considering conception, mature women and grandmothers and anyone who is passionate about conscious conception, pregnancy, birth and parenting. It will enhance your emotional wellbeing and move you towards a deeper understanding of your internal world. It provides empowering tools, fun and playful exercises and plenty of information.

By harnessing the creative process, it is possible to release buried thoughts and feelings that may hinder the natural flow of pregnancy and birth, and allow them to gently come to the surface and be expressed in a safe non-judgemental way. May the contents of this book encourage personal change so we can begin to create a new birth model by raising the consciousness that birth is the most fundamental experience of our lives.

⊥ Birth matters and what you think also matters

My journey to Bali, Indonesia, in 1998 was the catalyst for this book. Since then I have explored many aspects of birth, read extensively on Pre and Perinatal psychology from leading experts in the field, leaned from my practical experience with clients and groups, healed my own personal birth story and share my experience of the birth of my son. My research is underpinned by the marriage of two cultures, East and West and has enabled me to gain a deeper understanding about being a woman in today's world where conception, pregnancy, birth and motherhood have become a controversy. My work with women has allowed me to witness how, through the use of expressive art and personal exploration, they achieve deeper personal insight that has in turn made their pregnancy and birth more fulfilling.

Here are some of the areas we will cover:

- We will explore ways to have a more pleasurable conception, pregnancy and birth

- The Art of Birth – tools for empowerment to clear the way

- Fun creative exercises, visualisations, journal work, poetry

- The importance of fathers, partners and supportive relationships

- Positive Birth Stories and their power to heal and inspire

- Healing our own birth

- Reclaiming our true female power through birth

- Affirmations for birth – what you think matters

- History of birth psychology

- The Goddess within

- Feminine Sexuality (in its broadest sense)

- Spiritual pregnancy, birth and beyond using our intuition as guidance

- What to do if something goes wrong – looking at the bigger picture for support

- Find an independent midwife/doula/support who has a positive outlook of birth

The birth experience profoundly impacts both mother and baby. Although we may not be consciously aware of how our own birth shapes us, we are certainly influenced by it at cellular and unconscious levels. Birth creates a blueprint for our development. We take in an enormous amount of information during the first days and weeks of life, which in turn has a major effect on the ways in which we experience and respond to circumstances and people in our life.

↓ My body is safe, even though I may be feeling afraid (Binnie A. Dansby)

We have a large amount of technical/medical support for pregnancy and birth, yet offer very little emotional support for an expectant mother – and father. Pregnancy is a time of change in all respects, yet it is rarely acknowledged as being anything but a medical procedure. Research by leading experts such as Grantly Dick-Read and Sue Gerhardt, indicates that anxiety and fear during pregnancy not only affects the neurodevelopment of the foetus but also diminishes the mother's wellbeing and ability to give birth easily. What causes fear? It is usually fear of the mysterious power that surrounds birth, the potential pain and the many unfortunate stories about birth in our culture. We have, mostly, lost the ability to 'trust' our body/self and our intuition. I believe a woman will know exactly what to do if allowed to deeply trust the process.

↓ Whether you think you can or you can't, you are right

When we relax and trust our body, expansion is more likely and relaxation reduces pain. This sounds very simple in theory but if the general consensus is that birth is an ordeal, why would one 'relax'? Other contributing factors that may generate fear are previously unresolved traumatic births that become activated in subsequent pregnancies. Our own birth into this world will also be potentially activated in various forms; after all, it was our first birth experience. Most births are not given the reverence they deserve. Difficult life experiences may surface at this time and manifest as emotional obstacles, and yet there is no immediate support or outlet for these experiences.

Healing our life stories can have a hugely positive impact on our current birth. I know I would not be writing this book if it wasn't for all the support I received during my pregnancy, for all the art I made and how I processed my story. It was my most prolific time creatively and I produced extraordinary paintings which explored many of my unresolved issues... as I later discovered! I found making art was a spontaneous process and a great comfort that definitely supported my amazing birth outcome. Finding creative outlets to express any thought or feeling, however big or small, can really help free the way. If we take time to engage with our pregnancy and listen to our thoughts, we can work towards changing these thoughts from self-limiting to life-enhancing.

'Do the work you need to do on yourself. Our fears around birth can take over when we are in the altered state of consciousness that labour brings. It is essential to really get to the root of and clear these limiting thoughts, not just suppress them. When women are truly approaching birth from the right space, they tend to make choices that will support them.' (Roma Norris)

I have found that creative expression is the easiest and most pleasurable way to connect to our deeper selves and promote personal growth. We could say Art is a useful bridge between our internal and external worlds, with a concrete object as evidence. Art Making can be a fun way to explore our pregnancy while indirectly uncovering our inner world. It also offers us a constructive self-soothing 'time out' where we can tune into our baby and our body and receive its wisdom.

✦ Fear is created in the mind and can be resolved by the mind (B. A. Dansby)

In the West today, many midwives have had to become obstetric nurses who follow doctor's orders. Andrea Robertson, consultant in childbirth education and pioneer says, 'birth is a normal bodily function for a woman that requires a conducive environment and an experienced companion to watch for problems that may occasionally develop' (Robertson, A. 2002, Vol 5, No 7). Women possess ancient wisdom as birth keepers. Why are we not given more support and reverence as life givers? We all started life inside a woman and were born – even men! Many of us have lost our connection to the great earth mother who stands before us as an invisible but nonetheless powerful archetypal beacon. Carl Jung speaks of archetypes as being 'inborn forms of "intuition" which are the necessary determinants of all psychic processes'. They deal with the 'universal, inherited contents beyond the personal and the individual and they correlate with each other' (Hyde, M & McGuinness, M 1992).

How can we – women – believe once again in our own creativity and not fear our power to bring new life into this world? If we do not reclaim our body and our personal power we cannot blame the medical profession for taking over. According to Robertson, it is possible for most women (85-90%) to have a normal birth because nature has designed our bodies to do the job effectively. Nature sometimes has her own agenda which we cannot always change but by removing psychological barriers, we may prevent unnecessary complications. She believes 'birth is so safe and easy that almost always, any woman anywhere in the world, with no special education, training or experience, is capable of producing the next generation' (Robertson, A. 2002, Vol 5, No 7). She advocates that pregnancy and birth happen by themselves and so can birth, and that midwives are there to support the woman who inherently knows what to do. She argues that the natural pain of labour is essential and empowering, and promotes the home as the most natural place to give birth. Shiela Kitzinger says that 'the right place to give birth is the right place to make love' (Pre & Perinatal Psychology Conference, Toronto 1983). Home births are cheaper and there is plenty of research that shows how safe these are when compared to hospital births, with less intervention, less pain relief, virtually no separation between mother and infant post partum and lower mortality rate (British Medical Journal 2000, March 18; 320(7237): 798).

Additionally, the overuse of labour drugs, particularly in hospital, is greatly reduced with home births. Even though there is no evidence that any drugs are safe during pregnancy or labour, the first advice from hospital wards at the onset of labour is to have a Paracetamol and relax! (Haire, D. 1994 – cited in Robertson, A). I am not suggesting everyone must have a home birth in order to have a 'good birth' because it takes preparation and not everyone feels confident enough. If possible, you should give birth wherever you feel most comfortable and supported.

⚜ It is safe for me to feel all my feelings (B. A. Dansby)

We now have extensive evidence of prenatal memory and that the aural capacity of the foetus develops around sixteen weeks gestational age, which means that the foetus is able to learn from the senses (including taste and olfaction) as well as the emotional state of the mother and her environment (Chamberlain, D. B. 1998). The way in which we are born leaves an imprint in our body on a cellular level and on our unconscious. Dr Leboyer pioneered the idea of 'birth without violence' in the 1970's which compliments Chamberlains theory of 'traumas arising in the womb and at birth' (http://birthpsychology.com/person/david-b-chamberlain). Natural childbirth is less traumatic for baby and mother and leads to a more harmonious interaction. 'We must keep in mind that it is the child's first experience of life' (Dr Leboyer 1991, p140), so it is our duty to try and make this transition as easy as possible.

Pregnancy can be a time of great ambivalence. Joan Raphael-Leff puts it quite simply; 'To successfully negotiate the journey between being someone's child to becoming someone's parent, the pregnant woman and her partner, if she has one, will have to come to terms with mixed emotions and great shifts in the structuring of their sexual, couple, and personal identities' (Raphael-Leff 1995, p171). She emphasises the benefits of therapy or personal exploration during this time of great change because pregnancy can reactivate a 'past traumatic legacy' which therapy can help to work through. Prenatal therapy can also help to reduce 'the likelihood of postnatal depression and suicidal attempts, possibly preventing obstetric complications, and pre-empting the long-term effects of pathological parent-baby interactions, child abuse, and emotional neglect' (Raphael-Leff 1995, p171). 'There is evidence of increased incidence of anxiety and depression in pregnancy' (Gelder, N., Mayor, R., Cowen, P. 2001) and not just in the UK. However, the risk does not fall equally on all pregnant women. 'Mental disorders are more common in pregnant women who have a past history of psychiatric illness, family psychiatric history, past obstetric/gynaecological complications and C-section' (Scott, J., Jenkins, R. 1998). With these and many other possible experiences in mind, it seems vital that we treat the time between conception and birth conscientiously for all women in order to lay the foundations on which the future human being can grow, and to ensure a more pleasurable experience for the mother.

My Story

A Balinese Love Affair

My journey to motherhood triggered the writing of this book and enabled me to become a more conscious human being. My experience of pregnancy was shaped by two completely different cultures that compelled me to compare, contrast and create a new way of birthing that accommodated my whole being. I had just turned thirty and had split up with the man I thought was my big love. It was one of those 'turning points' in life and little did I know what was round the corner. I was living and working in London and struggling as an artist. My sister told me about a wonderful town in Bali inhabited by artists of all disciplines and gave me a Lonely Planet book. The pictures of Bali were the exact images of daydreams I had had as a child. So I decided to see for myself and went on a five week holiday to Bali in 1998 and immediately felt I had arrived home. After this trip I returned to England, sold my flat and I was back there in less than three months!

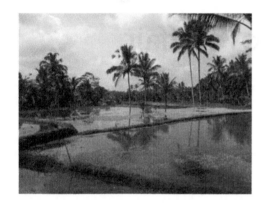
Beautiful Bali!

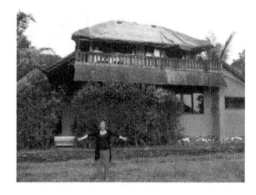
My first house in Bali re visited in 2009

I lived like a goddess and painted to my heart's content. My creativity flourished and before long I had created a large body of work and had my first exhibition in Bali which was received brilliantly. Artists and creativity are revered there; it is the foundation of their culture. There is nothing more satisfying, to fulfil your desires, than being respected, encouraged and celebrated for your creative achievements. I thought my dreams had come true – this was it! I then met the next 'man of my dreams'! He was a tall, dark and handsome Balinese who whisked me off my feet. The whirlwind romance was the talk of the town and we had the most stunning, exciting and extraordinary wedding imaginable. My husband really wanted to have a child with me and I became pregnant very quickly. This felt totally right at the time, despite the inevitable cultural differences between us. I was surrounded by positive energy that celebrated pregnancy, birth and motherhood as a valuable achievement. At a deep level this tapped into the core of my feminine desire to have children and be respected for this role. I had not experienced this feeling in the West and I think this is the reason why the feminine energy of Bali is so attractive to western women.

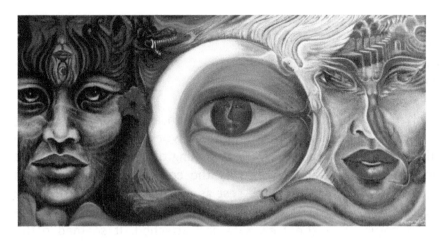

Moonlight Magic by Alexandra Florschutz 1999 (painted when pregnant)

MOONLIGHT MAGIC

(Poem by Alexandra Florschutz 1999)

Moonlight magic
Where dreams are made
Dark eyes feel
Through Marlborough haze.

Dazed hearts clear
Smoke screens lift
Pit of stomach falls
Let the dance shift.

Find no peace
Heat rising
Beating heart
Hunting the hunted.

Following footsteps
Yearn to be held
Playing the game
In love's shadow.

Lips meet lips
First time tremble
Hands wander
Clutching at straws.

Whole world sleeps
Fingers Dance
Smooth skin glistens
Bodies become one.

Dancing with Gods
Heaven paused
Rain falls straight
We fall in.

Melting moments
Then become three
Joyous second
Life-change forever.

Parting word
Kiss to you
Life to share
With one, not two.

Moonlight magic
Dreaming done
Fading sorrow
A new dawn has come.

Nights too short
When hearts pound
Undercover heroes
Breaking new ground.

I was deeply moved by the way pregnancy, birth and children were regarded in Bali. The spiritual connection with the 'unseen' world and nature allow women to trust in the process and treat the very beginning of life as sacred. Women aspire to become pregnant and are revered by the community. They look after their health, eat well, avoid stimulants, and rest as much as they can – even if at work, they go at a very slow pace. As soon as the baby is born she is held by the mother or family to ensure that she feels safe and attached. It seemed natural that I became pregnant there and felt very safe and secure. I had no tests, interventions or scans as I totally trusted my body and my pregnancy and it never occurred to me that I would need to have a doctor to tell me that everything was normal.

It is a Balinese tradition that the soul of the child comes from the Gods or heavenly realm and is protected by the Kanda Empat, or four siblings: the placenta, the amniotic fluid, the vernix caseosa and the blood. The relevance to the process of birth is described by Eiseman:

'...the *yeh nyom* (amniotic fluid) opens the door for the baby to exit, the *lamas* (vernix caseosa) and *rah* (blood) help on each side, and the *ari-ari* (placenta) pushes from the rear, coming out after the baby (hence ari – "younger" sibling). Of course, the fluid, blood and vernix disappear at once. Their physical remains are disposed of unceremoniously. The greatest attention, as described above, is paid to the *ari-ari*, since it is the only one of the four that is substantial.' (Eiseman, 1996)

It is important for the Balinese to acknowledge the four siblings as it is believed they hold much power and provide a connection to the spiritual world. The placenta is the most important aspect of birth after the child, as it is the only physical part that remains. Once a child has been born and the placenta delivered, the placenta is washed in water with a little turmeric, wrapped in white cloth or a palm leaf along with rice, special flower petals and some other symbolic items, and placed in a coconut shell. The coconut is then ceremonially buried in the garden outside the entrance of the main family home and a black stone is placed over the burial to mark the spot – which is to the right of the main front door if it is a boy and to the left if it is a girl. The placenta is blessed with daily prayers and offerings. This rite is to pay respect to the profound job of keeping the baby alive and nourished while she was growing in the womb. After every baby bath, the water is fed to the site and they sometimes add a drop of the mother's milk. It is also symbolic of the place where the child is born and secures it to her home roots.

No matter where the child is in the world later on in life, she always retains a strong connection to her home and family.

The Balinese believe that the four siblings have the power to keep the child safe, well and help her grow into a healthy adult. As Bali is a superstitious culture of folklore and symbolism, and their religion aims to keep the balance between the positive and negative forces in life, the Kanda Empat also have the power to bestow negative influences on the child if they are not properly respected. This encourages a conscious relationship between the physical world and the realm of the spirits.

The Balinese Ceremonies – Rites of Passage

I include the different Balinese ceremonial rites of passage which I personally experienced with my son, as an offering because it shows how a more spiritually-oriented culture approaches pregnancy, birth and beyond. I am also aware that other cultures have their own unique spiritual rites and rituals that support the journey of the human being.

The first ceremony is performed when a woman is around six months pregnant and definitely before she gives birth. The foetus is now fully formed and the four siblings are now present. The ceremony aims to purify the emerging little human being in the hope that she will grow up healthy, strong and live a meaningful life. The parents are encouraged not to use unnecessarily rough or inappropriate language and to be conscious of every thought and feeling as it is believed the foetus is tuned into the mother on every level, including her surrounding environment.

The second ceremony happens at birth and consists of the burial of the placenta outside the house, as I explained earlier. This ritual ensures that the Kanda Empat and the spiritual realms will support and protect mother and baby through what the Balinese believe to be a very vulnerable time.

The third ceremony happens when the umbilical cord falls away and the last physical remnants of the Kanda Empat are separated. The Kanda Empat now becomes more supernatural, like our spiritual version of a guardian angel.

Sometimes a ceremony is performed on the twelfth day to welcome the spirit of whichever ancestor has been reborn into the child, as they believe in reincarnation and the cycle of birth, life, death and rebirth. Twelve is also believed to be another sacred number in Bali and acknowledges the baby who now realises she is in a different world.

The first forty two days after the birth of the baby is called the *sebel* period and is a time when both mother and baby are considered 'religiously impure'. It is thought that the baby enters the world via the mother's genitals, where the blood and flesh and the physical earthiness of birth can attract unwanted spirits. These spirits, or *bujangs*, are shadow elements of the Kanda Empat that can threaten to lead the child astray. There are 108 *bujangs*, each related to a particular 'vice'. The mother does not enter the temple or perform any religious activity during menstruation or during the *sebel* period. When the umbilical cord falls off, the father is considered 'clean' again and the mother can enter the kitchen and cook. At the end of the *sebel* period mother and child are considered free from any dangers posed by the *bujangs*. I believe this is the way the Balinese 'give permission' to the mother to have complete respite after the birth and excuse her from her religious, cultural and gender specific duties! During this time she must remain in the family house/compound and do as little as possible other than care for her newborn. The mother and baby are protected in many ways by the father, grandparents and other household members. At forty two days, a ceremony is performed to mark the end of the *sebel* period.

The mother takes it very easy, resting a great deal and going about her duties in a slow methodical manner. Birth has always been a rite of passage for the mother who is conscientious about her role as bearer of new life. Once the baby is born she is held by the mother and later on by members of the family who never allow her feet to touch the ground, or leave her unattended until the first birthday which is called Oton in the Balinese calendar (a Balinese month has thirty five days, there are six months in a Balinese year which add to 210 days in their year). The first Oton is significant and so it is celebrated. The baby sleeps with the parents and is never without physical contact. As the child comes from the land of the gods, her descent onto the earth must be a gradual and respectful one. The mother stays at home nursing the baby with an un-phased, natural 'second nature' while the family members look after the mother's needs. The mother enables a secure attachment for the infant, caring for her every whim and the father/extended family encircles the mother and infant and looks after their needs. This support system ensures no one goes without care and support.

This picture ties in nicely with Attachment Theory, developed by John Bowlby. It argues that if an infant has formed a 'secure attachment' to the mother (preferably) or primary care giver from birth, who offers a 'secure base', then the child will grow up feeling much more supported and able to deal with life. (Bowlby, J. 1998).

The third Oton (about 630 days) marks the end of the ceremonies for the baby. The journey to earth from the land of the gods is now complete. The four divine guardians, Kanda Empat, have now become spiritually integrated within the body. They shave the baby's head to symbolise spiritual cleanliness and to celebrate the beginning of childhood. From now on, the annual Oton can be celebrated if the family wishes to do so.

At seventeen years old, the child has a tooth filing ceremony to mark the beginning of adulthood. The parents have paid everything up to this point and now it is time for the young adult to make her own way. The child will then pay for her children and so on. The child pays back the parents by organising and paying for their cremation ceremony.

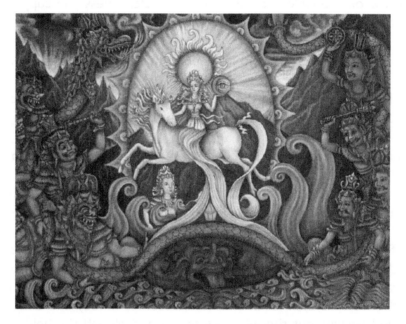

Tirtha Amertha (Elixir of Immortality) painting by Alexandra Florschutz

Balinese Ceremony Symbolism

I was fortunate to meet and get to know my son's grandfather and great grandfather. The great grandfather is a 'holy man' or Ducan with spiritual and healing powers. I talked with both of them and my husband on a sunny morning in their family compound in Pejeng. I asked them about the meaning of the many symbolic gestures that I witnessed during my son's birth ceremonies which I have summarised for your interest.

The ceremonies are performed in the home compound, usually in the family temple and adhering to specific codes of conduct. Sarongs are worn by everyone. The women wear a brightly coloured temple blouse (Kabaya), usually in a lace material which is see-through. They wear a sash (Anteng) around the waist and over their blouse. The sash is like a talisman to build your confidence and make you resilient to life's challenges, promoting diligence, not idleness. It shows respect for the gods, protects an important chakra and is part of the temple uniform.

During the ceremonies, the priest will often touch the third-eye area, shoulders, hands and feet with different objects such as an egg, a coin, a duck beak, rice, etc. The reason why the priest touches and blesses different areas of the body is thought to kill all the bad spirits inside it. The items used symbolise all that we wish to bestow on the child such as protection, cleanliness and support them to stay on the right path in life.

The egg has life inside it (Manik) and its symbolism is to keep the bad spirits away.

Coins are thought to clean out the bad spirits from the body. The coin comes from soft, rounded metal which, unlike a knife, is neither sharp nor dangerous.

Chicken and duck beaks are used in ceremonies to expel bad spirits. They symbolically guard the child in case someone tries to do something bad to her, like black magic. Chickens are considered holy animals in Bali and so are the duck and swan. These symbolise new life and enlightenment.

The priest first uses coins to try and locate bad spirits in the person's body and encourage them to come out. He then uses the duck beak to eat these spirits, in the same way that ducks clean up the rice field after the harvest (the rice is first harvested, the water is then let in and, as it becomes muddy and dirty, the ducks waddle around pecking out the leftovers to eat and plough the field at the same time leaving it ready for the next crop). The symbolism of the duck's beak in the ceremony is to find unhelpful energy in the human being and expunge it.

Rice is symbolic of the gods Brahma, Vishnu and Siva, and it signifies that the child will grow something in her life (Bija). You will often see a few grains of rice stuck to the forehead at the third eye point which usually suggests the ceremony is near the end.

A wool bracelet and subsequently a gold bracelet are placed around the baby's wrist or ankle. The significance of this is that they believe a child is born with nothing and must grow to find the treasure in her life. Gold represents the treasure that will come to her as a result of her work, and will not necessarily be handed to her on a plate. Sometimes the bracelets are taken off after three days but this is not compulsory.

Three coloured strands of cotton will be tucked behind the ears to show that the baby has already been through a ceremony and has changed as a result (banang). Also, as cotton can be straight and is natural, it encourages the child to do the right thing and always keep on the right path in life. Three represent the trinity of gods: Brahma (red), Vishnu (black) and Siva (white). The positioning of the gods in the temple is very important: Shiva is in the middle and represents Air, Vishnu symbolises water, and Brahma symbolises fire.

There is often a turtle drawn on the floor during ceremonies to symbolise the ocean and the support that the child will receive during her life.

The child is sometimes given a ring, a necklace and a headband as blessings from the priest and the gods.

Offerings of all descriptions, colourful and edible, will adorn the temple while a gentle, intoxicating smell of incense wafts through the air.

Grandparents also play a significant role by giving the baby money and are then allowed to hold the baby. Although the grandparent is related to the grandchild, they are far removed. They give symbolic money as a fast route to bring them closer together.

The grandchild, in return, is important and must be present at the grandparent's cremation as she is the one believed to allow the grandparents to go to heaven, the special place, paradise.

The Balinese see the human body as a container or 'box' which is inhabited by the immortal soul, *Atman*. They invite a baby into their lives and see birth and the early years as a time when the body and the soul are coming together. The ceremonies at this time support the process of embodiment of the soul in the body, its temporary home. Similarly, when a person dies, their soul leaves the body but is unable to return to god until they receive the cremation ceremony. The Balinese view of the world believes a human being is a microcosmic mirror of the universe. The body contains the five elements: earth, water, fire, air and space and must be returned to the macrocosm before the soul can be fully released from the body and make the transition towards reincarnation into a new form (Samsara). They believe the soul stays near the body it has just left until it is cremated and the elements returned to the universe. The soul may have an interim period where it experiences either heaven, hell or nirvana depending on its earthly behaviour. After the cremation, the ash is collected, taken down to the beach and released to the ocean. The body has returned to the earth/universe and the soul is set free to go on its next journey. This ceremony marks the end of the cycle of birth, life, death and allows the potential rebirth. I think this gives a lovely picture of how sacred the life cycle is to the Balinese and how important our entrance to life is from a spiritual perspective.

Story Continues – From East to West

When my husband was born at home, in Bali, he was placed in a palm leaf filled with warm water and colourful flower petals. The extended family surrounded him, sang gentle songs, and laughed and celebrated his arrival. In spite of hospitals also taking over in the last decade, this was such an amazing picture for me and remained like a beacon of possibility that I too might create a gentle, loving birth – the entrance to this life – for my own child.

All these ritual practices were at first fascinating and seemed too good to be true but something spoke to me on a deeper level. It presented the natural flow of life. The baby is conceived by making love, is nourished in a watery womb world of the mother's body and feels totally connected and loved, her needs being met without dispute. Then the baby is born into the world and instead of being separated, she is held close to the mother for as long as she needs. The wider family can take over as and when is required but the baby always has human contact. The child is then able to naturally take steps away from the mother because she has an innate trust in the Self and has a 'secure base' (Bowlby, J.) underpinning her emotional and psychological wellbeing. I believe this is why traditionally the Balinese children are so happy and easy going; they have not had to use their time and energy in self-protective mechanisms in order to survive. My experience of the way in which the Balinese relate to their infants, awakened my desire to raise my son along similar lines, by trusting my intuition. Unfortunately this picture is changing as Western practices take over from their natural methods and replace them with the idea that 'hospital is the safest option', where birth is a medical procedures. This is also now a big money making business at the expense of every family, until we change this picture!

The traditionally intuitive, secure, conscious way of pregnancy, birth and parenting is disappearing in the west and being replaced by an emphasis on the medicalisation of pregnancy and birth. Newborn babies are immediately encouraged (and this is almost at an unconscious level) to become 'independent' which is usually the result of corrective methods of withholding 'attention' which a baby internalises as love. The fundamental reason for this is fear that the child will grow up spoilt, needy and dependent on the parents. In my experience of the Balinese culture, providing a continual attachment does not create a problem.

There is a Balinese folk tale that celebrates motherhood in which the main character is a woman called Men Brayut, (meaning 'Mother of Many'). She has eighteen children and even though she is very poor, she and her husband Pen Brayut did an excellent job of raising their children. They would always listen to their needs, laugh and play with them and taught them by their good example. Their children grew up into remarkable adults who were known for their spiritual wisdom. The moral of the story is that proper child-rearing is the foundation of a healthy, balanced adult.

These ideas are not synonymous to Bali. Jean Liedloff describes in her outstanding book *The Continuum Concept* (2004), her time spent in the South American jungle with the Yuchana tribe. She observed how they raise their children with deep respect and care, providing a secure attachment as a continuum from the womb. The child gradually finds her own independence and all teaching, discipline, or 'child raising' is done by example with respect and love underpinning all. Liedloff later spent time researching the Balinese traditions and discovered that they too approached raising their children in a similar way to the Yuchana. I have only just read The Continuum Concept while I write this book and was pleased to discover that we both came to the same conclusion; that conception, pregnancy, birth and raising a child is a continuum of love, support and being present for your children when required. I feel that my original Bali experience is now being validated by Liedloff, an astonishing woman and author who dedicated her life to this research!

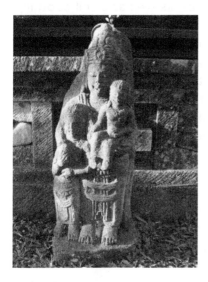

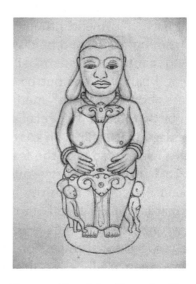

Balinese statue of mother & children   **Men Brayut** (sketch by Alexandra Florschutz)

I now knew how I wanted my child to be born and raised but events took another turn when we decided to move back to England when I was six months pregnant. I was met by a force field of negativity which quickly propelled me towards seeking an alternative picture. I researched a myriad of holistic approaches to pregnancy and birth. I joined a therapeutic birth preparation class, read many books, explored natural therapies, and found a support network. I was very lucky to stumble across a day conference in Brighton which offered a selection of the world's leading holistic experts in the fields of pregnancy, birth and parenting. I was particularly inspired by the work of Binnie A. Dansby, a gifted teacher, therapist, healer, author and philosopher with over thirty years experience supporting birth and who was the catalyst for my conscious, empowered journey to motherhood. Through her teachings, I received the clear message that pregnancy, birth and parenting could be a safe, positive experience if I engaged with the process. I received an empowered message through the ether, from the Balinese, that the cycle of life was safe, easy and a celebration, while I learned to actively engage with my inner world of thoughts and feelings and trust my own body's ability to birth my baby safely from Binnie's philosophy and other holistic points of view here in the west.

I joined a birth preparation class where I received support from a group of pregnant women, ran by Karel Ironside in Brighton (who is a wonderful SOURCE Breathwork Therapist, Active Birth Yoga teacher, Doula and mother), and worked on overcoming some of my newly emerging fears (especially my fear of caesareans) so that I could contemplate a home birth. To complement this I received one-to-one SOURCE Breathwork sessions from Pat Bennaceur, an exceptional therapist because I wanted to be as confident and free from unnecessary psychological and emotional barriers as possible. In addition to this, throughout my pregnancy, painting gave me the perfect channel for unconscious material. Expressing my creativity was often the best way of releasing past issues, as well as a self-soothing tool, and pure enjoyment! I thought I was 'OK' but it is interesting how issues can surface from one's past and be dissolved given the time and space. It felt important for me to educate myself on all aspects of pregnancy from a natural holistic standpoint. I balanced this out by doing the hospital tour 'in case' and went to an NCT class about 'pain relief' methods! Not once did they mention that a woman can give birth without pain relief and maybe even enjoy it! In Bali, I received the clear message that birth is an easy, natural and sacred rite of passage for women. In the UK, I was faced with the fear and negativity so often portrayed in the West – I was told that it was dangerous to have my first child at home even though I lived round the corner from the hospital. If something 'went wrong' it was highly unlikely that it would be fatal but they choose to focus on, and convey the 'what if it goes wrong' scenario. There is always a sad story somewhere and I have the deepest respect and compassion for that birth outcome but for most healthy pregnant women, birth can be straightforward.

In post war Britain of the 1950's, when health and housing conditions were fairly poor, women were encouraged to give birth in hospital because it was seen to be safer and more hygienic. By 1960 home births were at 33.2% in England and Wales and then rapidly declined to 2.5% by 2010. In the same period, caesareans rose to 25%; medical interventions 58% and 88.2% of births took place in a medical establishment (Office of National Statistics 2011). This does not seem like a particularly good advertisement for a Woman's most empowering and life changing rite of passage.

I have been researching natural birth for over a decade now and the more I look the more I find information that points to the fact that birth is easy and natural, albeit a full on experience. Birth does require one's whole being to harness our life energy and can be the most incredible experience a woman can ever have if she is supported in the right way. Even a caesarean can be a positive experience if the process is treated in a conscious and gentle way by the medical staff that are performing the operation.

➤ **It is safe for me to trust myself. My body is safe (B. A. Dansby)**

The Birth of Jude

I had the birth I dreamed of: natural, pain free, loving and peaceful in my own home. I awoke at 4.30am to a slight period-like twinge and when I went to the toilet I had the customary 'show' of blood. I felt a mix of fear (was there supposed to be so much blood? Maybe something was wrong?) And excitement ('this is it... show time'). I rang the hospital to register so they could send a midwife later. I was told everything was ok and normal, to take a Paracetamol and go back to bed. Now why would I want to take a drug that would go into my blood stream and into my baby – with all the nasty side effects that drugs contain – when I wasn't in any pain or discomfort whatsoever!?! I also wonder what implications labour drugs have on the baby, drugs for induction, epidural and anaesthesia for caesareans, and whether there is any link to problems which occur in children thereafter due to potent drugs entering their system at birth. Doctors emphasise the dangers of smoking, alcohol or drug use during pregnancy and yet the medicalisation of birth has become an accepted norm. So I avoided Paracetamol and just pottered about, went back to bed, rested, and later went for walks, climbed the stairs two at a time, ate nourishing food, did some drawing and listened to my empowering relaxation CD (called 'Having a Baby Is The Most Natural Thing In The World' by Binnie A. Dansby), in my birthing pool. If it is possible to have a birthing pool, then I totally recommend it – especially if you like water.

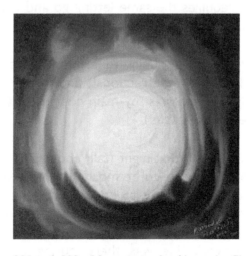

Watery Womb World – painting by Alexandra Florschutz

It was not until twenty hours later at 1am that the midwife arrived and until that time I was totally free from pain or discomfort. Between 1am and 4.27am the process gained momentum but it was nothing I could not handle. I had two painful contractions and this was because I was asked to lie down on my back for a dilation check – on reflection, a total waste of time as the baby was coming in his own time anyway. The second painful rush was when the midwife asked me a pointless question and jolted me out of my reverie! Never disturb a birthing woman! It was energetic, it took all my strength, I was tired yes (I like my sleep!) and it felt extremely powerful to be conscious of what I was doing every step of the way. I remember being slumped over the side of the pool, moving my hips from side to side and exhaling a deep guttural sound. The pool was in the sitting room and a dim light in the corner emitted a soft glow and I may have had some relaxation music tinkling softly somewhere. I was really tired and wondered if I was at the beginning, middle or near the end.

The midwife interrupted me at one point worried about how long I was taking and if I didn't hurry up she would think about transferring me! The audacity. She was, however, speaking from a place of fear and was trying to do her best. When she went out of the room I spoke to my baby and said to him "Hello my darling, we need to get you born..." And then there was a sinking sensation in my belly and the water's broke. My midwife came back into the room and checked the baby's heart rate which had increased slightly and she checked the broken water for Meconium. This is the first baby pooh which gets ingested by the baby during labour causing potential problems. Luckily it was ok and I think I told her I would like to be left alone. On my own again and all was well. I then felt a powerful need to push. It required a complete letting go of all resistance. So if there was anything I was still hanging on to... I had to let it go now! On later reflection, I sensed I had been holding on to self control a little because I was so used to this way of being. In the last hour or so the pushing was quite amazing and full on, like riding luxurious wild waves. It requires the same letting go and expansion like having an orgasm – you cannot hold on in fear and have a whole body orgasm.

I simply continued to focus on my belly, tune into the rise and fall of the body sensations (commonly known as contractions!) and do my best to flow with the intense energy. Wanting to sleep was my main concern rather than the so called pain (which was definitely manageable!)

My husband had a friend staying that night (talk about perfect timing) so he spent his time between us both. I wanted to be mostly on my own because I meditated through the process and did not want to be disturbed; he felt nervous and a bit helpless so his friend became a helpful distraction and support. Even though he came from a culture that considers birth easy and natural, he was still on his own without his support network. He was there during the last 'pushing phase', cheered me on and seemed to be in tune with what I needed. I had no interventions, no drugs or pain relief because I wasn't in what I would describe as pain, except for the four hefty pushes at the end to extract the head when I did feel a stinging sensation. I wondered if the head would actually come out and the midwives helped me to breathe and release the baby. This only took about ten minutes so it was bearable. (It was not any more painful than trying to extract a constipated pooh). I read this apt line in *Spiritual Midwifery*, 'Don't think of it as pain. Think of it as an interesting sensation that requires all of your attention' (Gaskin, I. M. 2002). I remember every detail with such joy and gratitude that I have always wanted to share my experience.

Nature is so much larger than we are and the energy is abundantly available for us to tap into during labour. We are invited to dive into the sensations we described as pain and surrender to this powerful energy, otherwise it will become about the pain and not about the flowing process, the rise and fall of rushes which pass through a woman during the birth of her baby. We need to deeply trust our instincts and override the cultural conditioning that teaches us to mistrust them. This is a time to be fully in the Feminine and cast aside the necessity to control, be goal oriented or prove one's equality to the Masculine – there is no need to be superwoman! A woman needs to be cherished, loved and honoured during labour by her partner and the caring birth supporters that surround her; and she needs to learn to receive this support. Also, slowing down in pregnancy and acknowledging the mind body connection can really help ease the stress of labour.

I believe I was empowered towards this achievement by exploring my internal world and expressing myself through art, positive affirmations and surrounding myself by people who trust the natural birth process. I believe everyone has the same chance to attract all the love and support available to be empowered givers of life, and to not be unnecessarily traumatised by a medical system, that does perform wonderful life saving work when needed, but does not always understand the meaning of natural and joyful Birth.

GIVING BIRTH

(Poem by Alexandra Florschutz 2000)

With belly full, I wait for you
Each hour could be the one
I take my breath into my heart
To open and become.

I focus far to outer space
From where we're made anew
I focus on you deep inside
Ready, waiting for your cue.

Relax, surrender to the flow
Our bodies knowing what to do
We are the mothers of this earth
Their lives depend on you.

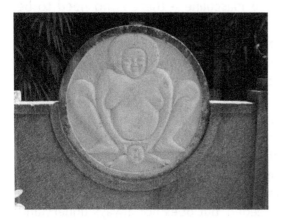

Bumi Sehat Birthing Clinic in Ubud, Bali
Founded by renowned midwife Robin Lim

Different Perspectives on Birth

General Literature Review

I have read extensively about conception, pregnancy and birth from many different angles including psychology, birth psychology, statistics from the NHS and other sources, art therapy, philosophy, art history, mythology, feminism and spirituality. The literature research, my practical work as an art therapist with women and my ongoing commitment to my personal development are the foundations for my work. The following authors have been of particular help in shaping my thoughts and this book.

Firstly, Clarissa Pinkola Estes who wrote *Women Who Run with the Wolves* (1998) totally inspired me as she describes how true feminine wisdom has been repressed for centuries and why women need to reclaim their intuitive power as 'Wild Women'. She describes fairy tales, myth and stories as a way of reconnecting to this 'wildish nature'; and through this, confirms the basis of my argument because pregnancy and birth is where a woman is able to tap into the depth of her being and bring a new life into this world. The woman is the authority during this time but many of us have lost our self-belief, intuition and trust in our body. Estes took me on a journey of self-discovery by weaving together story, interpretation and psychological knowledge.

Secondly, the philosophy of Louise L. Hay who wrote *You Can Heal Your Life* (2007) has helped me to understand myself and the way I think more deeply. Her life's work explores the identification of our negative core beliefs and how to change them to the positive truth. Negative thought patterns have been inherited from our childhood and the best way to clear them is by forgiving and letting go while affirming a new belief. Hay has also connected the way we think to the manifestation of illness or disease in our body. If we shift our beliefs, then we can change our physical wellbeing. It is really about taking responsibility for our life. This certainly helped me during my pregnancy because I was able to work on trusting my body and releasing my fears. She is a genius and a must read for pregnancy, birth and life.

Thirdly, the Archetypal Affirmations by Binnie A. Dansby work in a similar way. They become very powerful because they include a specific breathing technique which allows the release of our negative thought patterns buried deep at a cellular level. During the breathing session, the new positive thought is affirmed which becomes embedded in our consciousness speeding up the healing process. The affirmations can also be used daily to enhance well-being and prevent one from slipping back into old patterns.

Prenatal and Perinatal Psychology

Pre and Perinatal psychology explores the impact of our experiences in the womb, at birth and in the period shortly after birth. Even though most people cannot recall pre natal memories, these experiences do affect their neurological, biological and physiological makeup and reinforces the importance of care towards pregnant women and birth. Birthing with less intervention and pain, surrounded by conscious people who believe birth is natural, even ecstatic, is linked to happier and more peaceful babies. Dr Frederik Leboyer began to raise the consciousness of 'birth without violence' by asserting that the more gentle the birth the more happy the baby. Sheila Kitzinger, a leading authority on child birth, has been campaigning for decades to support the rights of the birthing woman who, she feels, gets swallowed up in the system and can emerge 'suffering from institutionalised violence' (Kitzinger, S. 2007). Michel Odent, a French obstetrician, surgeon and home birth midwife, instigated the ideas of the water birth pool and 'home-like birthing rooms' (Odent, M. 1999) in a state hospital. He argues that a woman needs to be in comfortable surroundings to allow her own intuition to guide her during labour and hence enjoy a more natural birth. The crucial time between birth and one year, he believes, lays the foundation for life. He highlights the importance of love and how it affects us at a molecular level. We find these themes mirrored by Sue Gerhard who has researched the profound effect that love and affection have on a developing baby's brain and nervous system. She describes 'how the quality of the relationship between parent and child influences both the biochemistry and the structure of the brain'. She argues that 'our basic psychological organisation is learnt from our generalised experiences in the earliest months and years' (Gerhard, S. 2004, p211), and in utero. The child will pick up repeated parental behaviours that will begin to write the baby's neurological script and over time become more of a permanent feature. Subsequent relationships will be approached from these early learnt patterns. So, how we respond to a baby's demands will have an immediate effect in shaping her nervous system. Janet Balaskas' Active Birth Movement in the 1980's advocated water births as being more gentle and trauma free for the baby - and mother. The report of a 1994 confidential enquiry by The National Birthday Trust Fund, which did extensive research into hospital versus home birth, found that there was a statistically higher rate of caesarean sections, assisted vaginal births and mortality in hospital than at home. Women found birth more enjoyable, felt more in control and felt less pain at home, yet hospitals are still promoted as the safer, more preferable option rather than the comfort and privacy of the home! I believe it is not so much about 'where' you give birth – there is nothing wrong with birthing in hospital, a birthing centre, home or other – but more about your own well-being.

⟟ A man is but the product of his thoughts, what he thinks, he becomes (Gandhi)

Alessandra Piontelli observed foetuses during pregnancy using the original ultrasound and continued observation after birth for up to two years. She concluded, unsurprisingly, that the experiences the mother has while pregnant – both psychological and environmental – affect the foetus. She provides evidence that this is noticeable during the child's development, which is to some extent predictable and she also concludes that a pre-birth attachment does exist. Piontelli proposes that the infant is already gaining experiences in the womb. Early research in Psychology believed that experiences began after birth and usually from the verbal stage onwards. John Bowlby argues for the importance of a healthy post-natal infant attachment to the mother figure for at least the first five years to promote balance in an adult. If the child is separated from his mother during this time it can have a devastating effect. There are arguments against this non feminist view but nevertheless a positive attachment needs to be made with a primary caregiver for healthy growth. Daniel Stern offers us a more scientific study on the 'development of the infant's sense of self' (2004). He found that the process of differentiation from the self and other starts from birth. He expanded the notion of whether difficult experiences in the pre-verbal phase of life would show up in areas of our life at a later stage. He thought that if we have a greater understanding of the way infants experience life, and consequently treat them with more sensitivity and respect, we might meet quite different adults in therapy.

Dr Lester W. Sontag wrote a paper in 1944 called *War and the Maternal-Foetal Relationship*. He observed that pregnant women with husbands at war were far more anxious and produced more unsettled babies. He speculated that the constant tension transferred from the mother to foetus would make the child 'emotionally volatile because his body machinery has been significantly altered in utero by an excess flow of his mother's neurohormones' (cited in Verny, T. 1981, p54). The child may later on create 'an emotional predisposition to anxiety' (p55). In England during World War II, Dick-Read (1944) also discovered 'that a tense woman had a tense cervix that impeded the process of her labour' which lead to his 'fear-tension-pain syndrome' theory (cited in Swan-Foster, N. 1989). Joan Raphael-Leff takes a more psychological approach and has thoroughly explored the inner journey of pregnant women from many different cultures around the world through psychotherapy. The diverse thoughts and feelings that emerged during the time of pregnancy found some solace in the therapeutic process.

The Holistic View

Binnie A. Dansby takes a holistic approach in her work as birth supporter, healer of traumatic birth experiences, teacher and visionary. She has created Archetypal Affirmations that help us turn our victim consciousness into creator consciousness. She promotes the powerful thought that to live in choice leads to self empowerment. Thoughts are creative: 'thoughts plus energy create results in the physical world', so it is important to pay attention to the attitudes that are present during pregnancy and at a birth as they all contribute to the outcome (Dansby, B. A. 1990). Her revolutionary work has expanded on the themes of Frederik Leboyer which forms part of the foundation of her philosophy.

'Birth is our 'Source' experience in our body, as we were conscious at birth and educable in utero. Birth affects our whole subsequent mental, emotional and spiritual well-being. It is the origin of our emotional response to every situation we encounter. The decisions we make at birth are the foundation for the beliefs and patterns activated in this lifetime. The quality of birth affects the quality of life and thus impacts and shapes the quality of society. We can easily see that the attitudes and patterns of each individual translate to the attitudes and patterns displayed by nations' (Dansby, B. A. 1998).

✦ A nation's culture resides in the hearts and in the soul of its people (Gandhi)

I found that the ideas of Rudolf Steiner, Thomas Weihs, Stanley Drake, and Bernhard Lievegoed, provided holistic and spiritual angles on pregnancy, birth and raising children. These schools of thought suggest a child comes from a universal spiritual dimension and incarnates into a personally crafted body with a potential set of tasks, or destiny to fulfil during her earthly existence. We must try not to interrupt this flow as much as possible.

Clarissa Pinkola Este's calls for the 'wild woman' to return to every woman and, through myth and fairy tale, find truth and empowerment. Anne Bearing & Jules Cashford, (1991), Arthur Cotterell & Rachel Storm, (1999), David Leeming & Jake Page and Larousse Encyclopaedia of Mythology (1959) gave me extensive insight into the history of mythology which allowed me to draw comparisons. Jung was my bridge between the mystical and the psychological. His theory on archetypes says that these are the essence of the collective unconscious and find a way of manifesting in many different guises, especially myth. If we are all connected on an unconscious level and we all possess a psychic part of ourselves that has the possibility to develop into deep intuitiveness, we can assume that what we think and feel can be picked up by others. We know this when we sense someone is in a mood with us and we can observe children picking up on our anxiety and acting it out.

⊥ Imagination and Creativity is the heart of humanity

It is therefore quite justifiable to assume that the mother's internal world is woven into the child's developing self. There is already so much research and evidence which shows the effects of separation and maltreatment of children, that it makes sense to examine the effects on the foetus in the womb. The Channel 4 documentary, Life before Birth (2005), used special camera equipment inside the womb to show the development of the foetus from conception to birth. We could see how the foetus responded to the external world in utero. This supported Piontelli's earlier argument. If we believe that we are able to pick up feelings and notions from the unconscious, like Jung suggests, and the foetus is educable in utero, then surely the foetus can experience the mother's psyche as well as being physically nourished by the connection of her placenta? This scientific research reveals how the complex interplay of our mental, emotional, physical and environmental systems influence the creation of a new human being. It highlights our collective responsibility, not just the mother's, to provide a safe, nurturing, loving environment for gestation, birth and life!

Art Therapy's Theoretical Base

Art therapists learn about all the different schools of psychology, and in particular the theories of Dr D. W. Winnicott and Wilfred Bion, who postulate the importance of a healthy mother-infant relationship for the human being to grow up psychologically healthy. Art therapy tries to simulate the essence of this theory and underpins our clinical practice. Bion postulates the notion of the mother being a 'container' who contains the infant's unbearable distress. What an infant projects out into the environment is gathered together and contained by the mother who soaks up the anxiety into her body, processes it and offers back the digested version. She has processed the child's fear and pain and made it more bearable. This gives the child the powerful message that she is not alone and separate in her task to integrate herself into her environment (Symington, J. 1996). Winnicott, on the other hand, suggests that the mother is a reflective mirror to the infant who symbolically 'holds' the child's distress helping her feel safe and protected. The infant sees herself in her mother's face which helps her develop a sense of herself. He thought that the interaction between the mother-infant relationship is a 'potential space' where anything is possible (Winnicott, D. W. 1971). The therapeutic relationship also tries to offer a similar experience for the client. The therapist is like the mother who tries to hold and contain the client's hopes and fears and reflect them back to be integrated in a more bearable way.

When we engage in expressive art, our unconscious thoughts and feelings are allowed to filter to the surface and become physically contained in the art object. Our experiences are then mirrored back to us for the purpose of further analysis, deeper understanding and healing.

Creation Mythology

World creation myths are mirrored in the conception of human life making pregnancy the ultimate creative process. Many cultures speak about the world being created out of 'nothing' or 'the primordial waters' of the universe by an omnipotent and often genderless god (i.e. the Book of Genesis), Egyptian, Australian, Greek and Mayan). Gods always had a female counterpart and vice versa and each had equal status and respect. Then there is life emerging from a world egg (Africa, China, India, South Pacific, Greece, and Japan) and Polynesians thought life was created from a coconut shell. In primeval mythology we always find a goddess whose sole purpose is bringing fertility, or being the archetypal mother. In Roman and Greek times we have the great mother of the triple goddess Hera and the earth/fertility goddess Demeter. The Celts had Dana the mother goddess and Brigid goddess of healing and fertility. Norse myth offers Frigg and Fjorgyn. Egypt, Mesopotamia and Iran have Isis (earth mother), Zarpanitu (birth goddess), Inanna (goddess of fertility) and Anahita and Tishtrya (water/fertility). In India and Japan are the mother goddesses from two different streams, Parvati and Aditi. There is also Gaia, Devi, Eve, Virgin Mary, Sophia and others (Cotterell, A., & Storm, R. 1999).

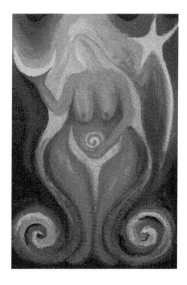

Moon Goddess – Painting by Alexandra Florschutz

One could also argue that there is gender equality. Where there is male, there is also female and neither can truly exist without the opposite like Yin/Yang. At conception the sperm meets the egg where it is fertilised and from the male and the female there is a possibility of creating new life. Polarities exist everywhere in nature like day and night; sun and moon, hot and cold. Life cannot be created without both genders – polar opposites.

I think the essence of mythology could reconnect us to something higher and more powerful than ourselves, instead of the current over emphasis of materialism. It suggests we belong to a greater creative source which may give us the strength to overcome our fear of giving birth and stay within our power. Women need to unleash the new 'Wild Woman' who, in the true words of Estes, 'are filled with passionate creativity, and ageless knowing; emotional truth, intuitive wisdom and instinctual self confidence' (Estes 1998). Women have traditionally been raised to keep their feelings quiet and be good little girls! So to achieve this inner freedom, or wild nature, we need to break the hereditary patterns that tie us to past ways of being. How can we do this? I believe it can be achieved by exploring ourselves creatively – to paint, draw, sculpt, dance, write, sing and express our truth – without agenda or judgement.

Your Feelings Matter

Emotional Support during Pregnancy works wonders

⚜ It is safe for me to express myself (B. A. Dansby)

Your feelings matter, that is the bottom line. If your feelings are validated and released you will feel better. In my experience, there are particular areas that would benefit from personal exploration before conception and/or during pregnancy in order to free the way from any emotional obstructions which might hinder the natural flow of birth.

- ⚜ Exploring how our own birth experience has shaped our life

- ⚜ Our previous birth stories with our own child(ren)

- ⚜ Reducing fear about giving birth

- ⚜ Working through loss and grief (i.e. miscarriage, ectopic pregnancy, still births, abortion, adoption and infertility, even caesarean)

- ⚜ How our past or current experiences can affect our well being during pregnancy, birth and the post natal period

The majority of pregnancies are normal, straightforward and 'low risk' and only a small number are 'high risk' due to health problems and given appropriate care. However, all human beings have been exposed to difficulties in their lifetime and yet we tend to either suppress or undermine the emotional affect these experiences may have on our well-being. Pregnancy, like menstruation, reduces a woman's ability to keep her emotional defences in place and instead she will conveniently, albeit unconsciously, manifest unexplainable emotional behaviour which she, or others, blame on her 'hormones'. By condemning a woman's emotions as 'hormonal', which equates to 'unimportant', she will immediately suppress them and lose touch with her most powerful navigational tool; her intuition.

Pregnancy is not always idyllic for some women but rather more intense. For example, if a woman is already in the care system she will more likely be offered psychological support which addresses not only her issues practically but hopefully takes into account her pregnancy. However, there are many women who may have had a range of traumatic experiences such as: miscarriage, abortion, sexual abuse, parental neglect, bereavement, loss, marriage problems, being a single parent, or a teenage parent, activated trans-generational trauma, etc, which can activate different symptoms during pregnancy. While pregnancy could precipitate a symptom like depression, for which help could be available, many women who may have had challenging experiences, unresolved issues, psychological problems or just day to day worries, have never found an outlet or resolution. They may be too nervous to address these unfamiliar emotions, or not conscious of the psychological influence their experiences have on their pregnant journey.

Clearing the mind of any subconscious emotional barriers to the smooth flow of labor (Gaskin, I. M. 2002)

⁛ I am the one who chooses what to think (B A. Dansby)

We experience a myriad of different thoughts and feelings during pregnancy – I know I did – both positive and negative. I struggled with my foreign husband as we tried to shape our cultural and religious differences and often wondered how my life would evolve. These thoughts and feelings are generally not talked about or given validation as 'normal' and ok to be expressed. I think, in general, we all feel that we have to put on a brave face and carry on. We may be in varying degrees of distress, develop post natal depression, problems with mother/infant bonding or pass unresolved issues onto our children. Ante-natal psychological support/therapy may not be an option, primarily because of the cost and because it is not readily available through the National Health Service or seen as an important part of the birth procedure to complement exercise (e.g. Yoga or Pilates), nutrition and medical support. Psychological/emotional support for pregnancy and birth should be available to all women should they feel they need it and I hope this book will be used as a self help reference book.

⁛ It is safe for me to feel all of my feelings (B. A. Dansby)

Some people are cynical about the idea that birth can be natural, gentle, trauma free, even relatively pain free. They expect it to be medical, painful, something to fear, blot out or anesthetise. But the more women, who do experience this positive possibility, make it more 'normal' for other women to do the same. Giving birth is an energetic process and fear is the most debilitating factor which impedes the natural birth flow.

⁛ Birth can be easy and natural

Fear and Birth

In the UK, medical interventions have reached an alarming 58% including the caesarean rate of 25% (around 50% in the USA) of which over half are elective caesareans (NHS statistics 2011/12). In a bid to reverse this trend, the Government has now 'recommended' natural birth as the preferred option to medically assisted births, as medical interventions are steadily on the increase and costly to the State (i.e. every 1% rise in c-sections cost the NHS £5 million – NHS

Statistics 2005). The data illustrates our increasing dependence on medical assistance in order to give birth. On the one hand we are told of all the dangers associated with pregnancy and birth and then expected to just have a natural one, so it is not surprising that women are disappointed when their desired outcome of a 'natural' or medically unassisted birth is not always achieved. It is not helpful that the media, soaps and films usually portray labour in an unrealistic, over-dramatised way, always showing the woman lying on her back in uncontrolled pain. Unless we change our collective consciousness from fear-based thinking to positive thinking about birth and refrain from portraying it in an inaccurate and dramatic way, we can then work towards creating more positive outcomes (i.e. normal, straightforward, even joyful births). I think only then will these statistics begin to decline.

How has birth become so medicalised? I think it has to do with several factors. Firstly, there is the emphasis on birth being a potentially difficult procedure which only medically trained people (and usually obstetricians who are male - in most cases) can undertake. We are never given the message that a woman's body knows exactly what to do and she can do it perfectly well if she has enough space and time and a supportive midwife/doula/partner/other. A midwife has been described as 'a wife to the mother' who 'stays with you through all your changes in labour and keeps believing in you' (Gaskin, I. M. 2002). If the expectation of medical intervention was less, then the majority of births could be natural. The Association for Improvements in the Maternity Services (AIMS) has great information about anything to do with pregnancy/birth at www.aims.org.uk, and an interesting article called Home Birth, The Normal Option: www.aims.org.uk/ Journal/Vol20No3/homebirthTheNormalOption.htm

⚜ Thoughts are creative so it is important to know that you are completely safe

Through my research I noticed that the medicalisation of birth appeared with the resurgence of Feminism in the 1960's, which campaigned for the rights of women to enjoy equality with men, be independent and make their own choices (which I'm totally for). Traditionally, babies were born at home but, as hospitals started to be advertised as the safest place to give birth in the 60's and 70's, they swiftly became the norm. By 1980, after the Peel Report, 'medicalised birth also became the norm' (Edwards, N. AIMS Journal, 2008, Vol 20. No 3).

I believe that birth has become a covert way by which the patriarchal system tries to control the Feminine by undermining a woman's intuition and her innate trust in the natural processes of her body. One of the contributing factors is making c-sections and epidurals appear a seductively preferable option masquerading as choice. I would like to clarify that I am not against caesareans or judge any form of medical procedure, as these can be lifesaving, but I am highlighting a growing problem which affects the mother's experience of giving birth. If 25% of all UK births are by caesarean and half of these are emergency, then there are still a significant number of elected caesareans performed for no emergency reason. We should also be asking why so many women are having such traumatic births which often result in an emergency caesarean that may have been prevented under the right circumstances and what can be done to increase the number of natural births. This trauma not only affects the mother but has a significant impact on the infant. (Post Traumatic Stress Syndrome, PTSS, has been linked to the experience of a traumatic birth).

At a time when births are often described in a negative way (usually because they have been very difficult), it is not surprising that women opt for a procedure which advertises safety, efficacy and the potential absence of pain. We prefer to choose a medically controlled operation (major abdominal surgery) where we believe we are in safe hands, instead of venturing into an unknown realm of unnecessary pain. Women often feel it is their right to opt for a total pain free birth by epidural and/or c-section. It is still handing over our power to an unnatural process, which poses health risks, instead of taking our bodies into our own hands and riding the waves. I think true feminism is daring to journey into this unknown realm of birth and be the mistress of our body, mind and intuition and not willingly hand it over to a system that thinks it knows better. Our bodies were designed for birth, so it is better to get reacquainted with our precious bodies as they hold all the information we need. Let us change the self-fulfilling prophecy that 'birth is a painful, nightmare experience' because that is what will continue to happen if we don't change our minds and free the way.

..taking our bodies into our own hands and riding the waves

Any form of medical procedure in an emergency situation or due to health risks is totally justified if it saves the lives of the baby or mother - it is important not be too rigid. It is when caesareans become routine that we perhaps need to ask why. However, if you desire a caesarean for whatever reason, then it is possible to create a positive experience, even in an emergency. For example, you can inform yourself about the procedure, ask the staff to play soothing music, keep voices low and respectful, have your partner or a supportive person with you during the operation, ask to watch the delivery (by lowering the curtain so you can see your baby), ask for immediate skin to skin contact and ask the staff to support breast feeding as soon as possible. There is more useful information at these two websites:
http://www.birthrites.org/caesarean.html
http://www.birthcut.com/thepositivecesarean.htm

I would like to see the world of birth become a life-enhancing and empowering place rather than being driven by fear and control.

I think most women are afraid of actually giving birth whether this is conscious or unconscious. I know I entered the realm of fear on my return to the UK which I strived very quickly to resolve. This fear has a profound effect on our body. To give birth 'naturally' one needs to enter into a 'primal' state of being. During labour, our intellectual brain (neo cortex) switches off and we drift into our primal brain or state. If this state is interrupted, it can prompt the slowing down of contractions and alarm the medical professionals. This state is very often interrupted when electronic monitoring gadgets such as Electro Foetal Monitors are used and these have been strongly linked to the rise in c-sections (NHS Statistics). Relying on an electrical gadget to tell us how a woman's labour is progressing is very different from a woman feeling comfortable with her body's progress. Also, it is all very well saying women need to immerse themselves into this primal, dreamy, in-focussed state but we don't live in a society that allows for any time to reflect, slow down, or look inside, unless one does it consciously. To be sufficiently engaged in this primal state one must relinquish one's self control and revel in this 'other world' state of being. The mind plays a large part, so if we believe birth is painful and difficult then it will be, but if we only have heard horror stories then how can we possibly think it would be any different? We lead fast pace lives, seldom stopping to relax and prepare and then we expect to just slide into a primal state of being when labour begins. I think this is unrealistic without any preparation during pregnancy. An athlete would not run a marathon without adequate mental and physical training. Nor can we expect a woman to birth a baby without some kind of psychological and physical preparation beforehand. Acknowledging the emotional lives of all pregnant women, spring cleaning our histories before the birth and addressing any new fears, worries or anxieties that may arise, can really help free the way and support an easier journey through pregnancy, birth and beyond. It is a time of celebration!

The potential benefits of this preparation include: normal birth, less medical intervention (i.e. caesareans), the reduction of the need for drugs, shorter labour, increase in breastfeeding, the reduction of incidences of post natal depression, better mother and infant bonding, a more positive experience for both the mother and baby and a positive impact on society.

It is safe to take full deep breaths (B. A. Dansby)

I think the use of art as a therapeutic form of self expression is highly compatible with the creative process of pregnancy and birth. It offers a route to unconscious feelings, allows one to experience 'mess', is fun and self soothing and does NOT require any skill whatsoever!

Unfortunately, nowadays birth and motherhood is perceived as unimportant and inconsequential. The current trend aims to define women by their careers and having a baby is often seen as a mild inconvenience. I wish to inspire you to trust your body and open your mind to the concept that being a parent is the most valuable job in the world. Most importantly, there must be no blame towards the mother for any birth outcome but an increase in the support and positivity that surrounds her so that more women having positive experiences can act as beacons to balance out the current fear-based approach so rife in our culture.

✦ I am loved and accepted exactly the way I am (B. A. Dansby)

I think this next passage from *Spiritual Midwifery* by Ina May Gaskin (2002) expresses very beautifully the importance of creating a positive atmosphere to promote endorphins which make labour much easier.

'I believe that much of the reason why the women whose births we attended were able to get through labour without anaesthesia or tranquilizers had to do with the atmosphere we learned to create at a birth. There is a sound physiological explanation for why some women experience more pain in labour that others. A woman who is the centre of positive attention, feeling grateful, amused, loved and appreciated, has a higher level of the class of neurohormones called endorphins. Endorphins actually block the perception of pain.

On the other hand, there are also adrenalin-like substances which may be secreted by the body during labour, especially when the woman is afraid, cold, angry, humiliated or experiencing any other disagreeable emotion. Adrenalin is part of the body's protective mechanism when it is presented with danger; the heart rate quickens, the muscles tense, labour contractions may be inhibited, and the perception of pain is intensified. The mother is made ready to fight or to flee when adrenalin levels are high, not to have her baby' (Gaskin, I. M. 2002).

Creating a positive, supportive, humorous, loving environment at birth – which one can begin to create in the home during pregnancy – will increase endorphins and make the birth more enjoyable. Fathers can play a really important part during pregnancy and birth by allowing and validating their pregnant partner's free expression and this also applies to same sex partners. By being loving, caring and listening, really supports the mother-to-be. A man has his own journey during pregnancy and this process has generally been undermined also by the medicalisation of birth.

Fabulous Fathers

Support, support, support! Fathers can really help a birthing woman by being present, loving and supportive. Gentleness, touch, love, kisses, hugs, nurturing, intuitiveness are all qualities that a partner can develop to support the mother. This is also relevant to partners in same sex relationships. Often a man can feel 'left out' and helpless during labour and clicks into his Mr Fix it mode. It can be very scary for a man to stand by and watch his beloved writhing around in what looks like unbearable pain and making animal-like noises. This is a normal expression but it can sometimes be more pronounced if she has been induced or given drugs. He wants to make it all better and, without understanding the powerful sensations of labour and that a woman needs to express ALL of her feelings, he will do everything to put an end to her suffering – even if this leads to a caesarean. The fear he experiences is understandable and he is also having his own unique journey from conception, through pregnancy and on to birth.

There is hardly any literature out there that talks about the father's journey! He is half the equation and has helped create the child, even though he does not physically give birth to his child, he will give birth emotionally. Hence, the best thing a father can do is find his own support network, do his own inner work, process his own birth into this world and then be a balanced container for his birthing partner. Communication beforehand is paramount so he can be even more in tune with his partner and hopefully intuit her signals during labour. Fathers may work through most of the creative exercises in this book, keep a journal and also do the centring process because the more relaxed and 'in his body' a father can be, the more energetically supportive he will be for his partner.

+ **The most important thing that a father can do for his children is to love their mother (Hesburgh)**

Affirm feelings of safety for both yourself and your partner: 'My body is safe', 'my partner's body is safe' and 'my baby is safe' are all useful affirmations. For more in-depth support for fathers read the *Fathers-To-Be Handbook – A Road Map for the Transition to Fatherhood* by the renowned Patrick M. Houser (www.fatherstobe.org). Patrick's quest is to enlighten the collective nature of the time between conception and birth in family life, in particular by the inclusion/participation of the dad.

How the Balinese do it

This section is really for your interest and not to suggest you simulate the Balinese traditions. Although I have mentioned some of their cultural ways earlier in the book, I wish to elaborate on it further. The Balinese treat conception, pregnancy and birth, like all important life events, with great reverence and respect. The religion is unique, a combination of their version of Hinduism with elements of Buddhism and Animism and Sang Hyang Widhi Wasa as the supreme God. Out of this spiritual wisdom emerged the ceremonial rituals which help to maintain the positive and usually happy outcome. These attitudes support the pregnant woman and seem to create happy balanced children as a result. In the West, we could greatly benefit by re-learning to respect the sanctity of the beginning of life in order to tip the balance back in favour of a more pleasurable experience. The entrance to life is a momentous event, so ensuring it is a gentle, conscious passage is much more desirable for the new human being – just as the end of life, our death, should also be treated with the same love and respect.

I therefore, wish to share with you how the Balinese approach conception, pregnancy and birth both in ritual and philosophy as I think it gives a wonderful picture of how a whole culture honours this process. Although the ideas may seem radical or farfetched, they all support this rite of passage so beautifully. It is certainly what inspired me to 'dare' to become pregnant surrounded by people with whom I felt safe and respected. In the UK I always felt that 'work' and 'career' were more important than motherhood (my thought pattern, I know, but I am aware that it is quite a common one!) and so the experience of motherhood was always postponed. I am certain this is why many western women, who find their journey leading them to Bali and such places, are seduced by the devotion of the men who believe marriage and children far exceed career in terms of importance. The men genuinely really want to marry and are very excited about creating a child, not just for the fun, but because it is part of the natural birth, life and death process of life.

Conception: The 'Balinese tradition' recommend having sex on an auspicious day according to the specially prepared Balinese calendar which originates from the Lontar – the holy tradition handed down through the ages although its beginning is unknown. It is connected to astrology and worked out in a rather complicated and convoluted way. A person can even use it to check whether it is ok to visit a relative on a certain day, get married or build a house! A calendar is produced every year with information the Balinese follow religiously. And sex in the afternoon when pregnant is not recommended for some reason! I never found it a problem though!

⚜ I am connected in love to all that lives and all that breathes
(B. A. Dansby)

Diet is very important and pregnant women are urged to refrain from eating pork, eel or any meat because of the association with the animal energy. The idea is that anything the woman takes into her body has an influence on the developing embryo so they avoid alcohol, tea, coffee, fizzy drinks, stimulants, toxins, or unhealthy food. Even cuddling animals like cats and dogs is not encouraged!

They aspire to become conscious of what they do or say, try to keep their thoughts positive and their emotional life balanced. Ideally they practice yoga, pray daily and try to stay happy which they believe will support a good birth and create balanced children. This is what one tends to experience in the Balinese children. Also, the pregnant woman does not go to a wedding ceremony as this might confuse the embryonic development with the wrong ceremonial messages!

At seven months the embryo is completely formed into a baby and a ceremony is performed to thank the gods for forming the baby and ask for a good, safe birth. The Kanda Empat (four siblings) are also asked to protect the process from womb to birth. They are part of the 108 'family members' that 'live' in every human being's body and relate to every part of the body (skin, blood, teeth, etc) with an individual name. So if a person e.g. has a headache, the family member connected to the head is treated! As previously mentioned, the four siblings correspond to the placenta, blood, amniotic fluid and vernix caseosa. The 'family members' have a contract with the new human being to bring her down from the gods to the earth and remain with the baby until three months after the birth (105 days). After three months the baby 'forgets' her family members and they depart one by one back to the realm of the gods. The Kanda Empat remains with the child for around eighteen months, as previously described.

⚜ I am open to receive all the love that comes to me
(B. A. Dansby)

Once the baby is born, usually at home (although this is changing to simulate western methods), the baby stays attached to the mother all the time. Ceremonies are given at days 3, 12, 42, 105 (3 Balinese months) and 210 (6 Balinese months or 7 western months). The six month ceremony, or first Oton, is the child's first birthday according to the traditional calendar. There is a ceremony for the second Oton and the third Oton (about 18 Balinese months) marks the end of the first stage of life. (Other ceremonies take place when the teeth begin to appear, when the last milk tooth falls out, at puberty, tooth filing to 'tame the wild element' in the person, marriage and lastly, the cremation ceremony which completes the cycle of life). These rituals provide the space and time for the family to consciously welcome the new child. They have the opportunity to recover and adjust to the new arrival and allow the woman to really be looked after and freed from most of her responsibilities other than caring for her new born. Life is a conscious process.

Can you imagine the West translating these methods into our life? I know there are growing communities who do honour the life of the human being but we are still in a minority. How wonderful it would be for a baby to enter the world surrounded by conscious people and be honoured every step of the way? Or when our daughter starts her first Menses and is celebrated for the fabulous woman that she is transforming into during adolescence? And our son honoured for his power and gentleness to go forth into the world and share his gifts in a safe and inspired way? I think these cycles would help us to 'enjoy' the rearing of our children once again before our busy lives take over completely. I believe parenting is the most fulfilling, life enhancing, transformative job in the world and can also be the most challenging! Maybe we need to find a renewed way of balancing our career and raising our children.

The Art of Conception

The Magic of your Thoughts

Your beliefs become your thoughts
Your thoughts become your words
Your words become your actions
Your actions become your habits
Your habits become your values
Your values become your destiny
(Mahatma Gandhi)

In this chapter I would like to offer some insight into the power of our consciousness and how as parents we are co-creating human life. This is particularly relevant to conception (and even pre-conception). There is much debate about nature versus nurture; are we a product of our genes? In which case parenting has little consequence other that common sense care, or is it down to our environment to affect the outcome? Well, according to Bruce H. Lipton and others, '...parents have overwhelming influence on the mental and physical attributes of the children they raise.' (Verny and Kelly 1981 cited in Lipton 2009). And apparently this all begins before birth!

It is thought that the environment, created by the parents, not only affects the development of the child (both pre and post birth) but contributes to genetic determination. Many leading experts in the field of pre-birth life (Thomas Verny, David Chamberlain, Dr Peter W. Nathanielsz and many more) emphasise the importance of creating a nurturing and life-enhancing environment for the developing foetus which will assist a lifetime of better health. It even enables the brain to grow more healthily because the right genes have been activated by this environment. The following quote explains it clearly,

'The responsiveness of individuals to the environmental conditions perceived by their mothers before birth allows them to optimize their genetic and physiologic development as they adapt to the environmental forecast. The same life-enhancing epigenetic plasticity of human development can go awry and lead to an array of chronic disease in old age if an individual experiences adverse nutritional and environmental circumstances during foetal and neonatal periods of development.' (Bateson, et al, 2004, cited in Lipton 2009).

This is not meant to incite guilt but rather, once we understand that what we do as parents really matters, then we have the choice to make that extra effort to provide a holistic environment so our children will reach their full potential. Naturally, we have inherent behavioural instincts which are nothing to do with where, when or how we were born and yet we learn how to respond to these natural behaviours from our parents. As children take in their surroundings, they will subconsciously adopt their parents' ways and beliefs which may look as though it is genetic. It is a kind of 'brain washing' which can be either positive or negative.

I think it is important to add that when we have a child, our circumstances are unique to that child at that time which will be different to subsequent children. There are not one set of parents who are the same as another. We are individuals who have been raised uniquely. I would like to take it a step further and suggest that each human being has a 'soul' that is their absolute own and not like any other person's. The soul contains the imprints of the experiences of many lives, like our very own suitcase with our particular contents. Rudolph Steiner has described us as complex spiritual beings that come to earth to have certain experiences, to learn, to give, to develop and we chose our family constellation and culture in order to support this growth. He also describes our four interactive 'bodies': Physical, Etheric, Astral and Ego (our Higher Self, not to be confused with ego or egotism). If these bodies work in harmony with each other then the physical and emotional wellbeing of a human being is healthy. Naturally, the environment and the genetic makeup of the person will also affect this harmonious interplay of the different bodies.

So, if we consciously provide the best foundation we are able to offer at the time, and are willing to learn as we raise our children – I know I have had to adapt significantly to support my son's needs – then that is sufficient. We cannot, however, prevent our children from having experiences which, in the long run, may benefit their personal development and have nothing to do with how well we parent. For example, we may have done all we can to prepare for a straightforward birth but for some reason the birth has had its own plans, nature has decided her way. Or a child may have an accident which enables the family to change direction or have a learning experience or even help others. Of course we would not wish anything on our children but an empowering view of the situation can help tremendously.

Perhaps we can surmise that having a baby is an amalgamation of genetic inheritance, or evolution and epigenesis, the uniqueness of the individual on which the environment has an important influence. Both of these theories are contained within the human soul – the individuality which pertains to each human being – their deepest essence which has lived for many incarnations within many different physical bodies. These theories and ideas can be read in many wonderful books, including Rudolph Steiner's timeless natural scientific research, or revealed through meditation.

If we return to conception, then it is really valuable to invite into our consciousness the concept of how powerful our mind and intentions are and their general effect on our health. There is much research taking place which validates this notion and most people know of the placebo effect in medicine. If you believe you are being given a life saving treatment, your innate trust in its efficacy potentially allows you to heal. In contrast, there is also the nocebo effect (nocebo means 'I will harm' in Latin) where the 'reaction or response is the harmful, unpleasant, or undesirable effects a subject manifests after receiving an inert dummy drug or placebo. Nocebo responses are not chemically generated and are due only to the subject's pessimistic belief and expectation that the inert drug will produce negative consequences. In these cases, there is no "real" drug involved, but the actual negative consequences of the administration of the inert drug, which may be physiological, behavioural, emotional, and/or cognitive, are nonetheless real' (http://en.wikipedia.org/wiki/Nocebo) .

We could argue that this theory applies to pregnancy and birth too and I hope encourages you to work on a positive mental outlook as much as possible. This is why fear and anxiety have such a massive influence on our health and wellbeing which in turn will contribute to the outcome of our birth. Fear and birth are not compatible.

Conception can be planned or left to fate, let's see how it goes. Even if it is an unplanned 'accident', we can start to think about the potential of this human being which has come to us in order to experience life. I invite you to think about conscious conception as a legitimate option and to focus on the responsibility you have for this new life – which by no means, excludes revelling in wanton ecstasy. It can be such fun to honour the potential of your baby, like the Balinese do, with ritual, song, prayer, meditation, communication, art and above all, if possible, joy. If conception was unplanned and you are frightened and unsure, then working through some of your feelings will help to clear the way. I offer lovely art exercises for you to do later on in the book which allow your creativity to unleash the potential for ecstatic conception.

⚜ Life only produces life (B. A. Dansby)

The conception of my baby was a very complex and unusual experience, in my opinion. I had a very strong sense that I had to be in Bali; it was as if a powerful hand was guiding me there and a strange turn of events allowed this to happen (that is another story). I was not considering a relationship with a culturally different man but one night, through the haze of a smoky bar, there appeared the most gorgeous man I had ever met. It really was love at first sight although he was not what I imagined as a husband or father figure for my child. Nevertheless, the feelings were mutual and he wooed me into marriage and, after one night of wanton abandon and no protection, I knew I had conceived. I had the feeling our relationship would have its set of challenges but something deep inside gave me the courage to continue – although had I known what the future held, I might have reconsidered. In retrospect, even though my birth was extraordinarily straight forward and enjoyable, the journey since birth has been extremely challenging and yet I would not exchange it for anything. I believe it has made me a much deeper, more interesting and compassionate person than I would ever have been had I not manifested this story. If your parental journey has had a similar beginning then embrace the future with open arms and learn from your story. I often wonder whether it was 'my destiny or fate' that brought us together or if it was due to my unconscious behaviour and fear that I blindly allowed myself to enter into the relationship, marriage and conception. And yet had I not had the whole experience, I may not have been desperate enough to develop myself and transform the challenges into a positive future with my son. This book would not exist either! Today, I see it as a karmic deal between my son's father and me and that we both have had our unique journey. He has had the chance to develop himself here in the West, work, be a father and support his family back home in Bali while I have had to learn to grow up and be responsible. I now understand that all actions have consequences and that we make choices we have to live with and embrace.

The Art of Birth

Expressive Art for Self Development

The Art of Birth is a supportive way to explore your inner world before, during and after pregnancy using Expressive Art. Expressive art means that you use art materials to express your thoughts and feeling without having to make a 'good' picture. Through creative, fun and playful exercises, based on the principles of art therapy, you will be able to deepen your experience of birth. Our thoughts and feelings have a direct influence on our physical body and health so it can be helpful to release any emotions that may inhibit the natural process of birth. Self expression through art offers a powerful tool for transformation when words may not be enough. Most people think they are not creative, or say they were not good at art in school. You may even feel inhibited to do the creative exercises but once you are given permission to 'go for it'; you will be surprised at the outcome. Anyone can be creative and no experience of art is necessary as it is not about technical skill but creative freedom. We have the opportunity to experiment and make our own creative decisions or test drive ideas. Once we have an image in front of us, it allows us to reflect on what we have created as we have physical evidence of our expression. Pregnancy and birth can be a profound rite of passage for a woman. The essence of child birth preparation is self discovery, so you can give birth in awareness. It is not necessarily about trying to achieve a specific birth outcome. Please note that there is no judgement towards any birth outcome as this is more about supporting the process through self development.

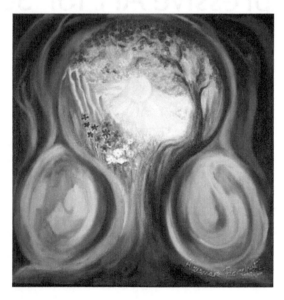

Womb Paradise – painting by Alexandra Florschutz

The Art of Birth offers you the opportunity to

🖊 Explore the process of pregnancy and birth creatively

- Look at your own birth story

- Enjoy playing with different art materials (experiment with colour, line, shape, texture and symbols using paints, pencils, pastels, clay and mixed media)

- Allow yourself to make a MESS as birth is generally messy

- Use art as a form of expression and transformation

- Express feelings honestly and spontaneously and work through any issues to gain greater self-knowledge

- Dispel the myth of fear surrounding birth

- Explore the possibility of an ecstatic birth

- Rejoice in connecting with yourself and your baby

- Interpret your art work to see what it can reveal to you

Whether you are in a group or creating at home by yourself, have fun playing with the materials and allow free range to your imagination.

'It's not about being good enough or about being a professional artist. It's about finding the images within your imagination, your soul, and then loving and honouring them by painting or sculpting or drawing them into creation. Bring your images into the world as you would bring a child into the world' (Rominger, J. 1998 cited in *Birthing from Within*).

The Amazing Benefits of Art

Art and birth have been major parts of human life since the beginning of human evolution. We are all aware of the Palaeolithic pregnant figures carved in stone that are thought to represent female fertility and the Sheela Na Gigs, which are carved squatting female figures with exaggerated vulvas, mainly found in Ireland and some parts of Great Britain, at the entrance of churches, castles and buildings. They are thought to provide protection, represent fertility and the mother goddess in the pre Christian era. More recently, the artist Frida Kahlo used painting to express her traumatic experience of pregnancy and miscarriage, a subject that is rarely portrayed in art. Creating art and creating a human life can be seen as parallel achievements of enormous significance to a woman.

⚘ Art is a powerful form of expression

We can use art as a way of communicating our thoughts and feelings without having to use words – a kind of symbolic speech – because it has the ability to access the 'unconscious' part of ourselves. This is where we bury our pain, hurt, frustrations, anger, fears and difficult memories especially from childhood, birth or even in the womb.

Art inevitably tells our personal stories about our feelings, thoughts, experiences, values and beliefs. In the process of making these visible through art, we are offered a way to know ourselves from a new perspective and an opportunity to transform that perspective. There is no pressure for technical skill or having to produce a beautiful picture, in fact, no experience of art is necessary, just a willingness to have a go. A wide variety of art materials and mixed media are available nowadays at a very low cost which we can use in a free way – any mark is a valid contribution. Often we find symbols emerging over time that have a particular relevance to our lives, or a single image that can speak volumes.

Aim to create an environment that is at all times safe, nurturing and free from interruption if possible, for you to experiment and play with the different art materials. This kind of environment will provide security for you to express feelings honestly and spontaneously and work through any issues to gain greater self-knowledge. You can learn to explore and interpret your own art work to see what it might reveal to you. This contained freedom can be very liberating. If you have other children or a toddler then you will have to make suitable arrangements to create a space for yourself. Otherwise it may be easier to write and draw in your journal so that you are able to express your thoughts and feelings more immediately.

(In an Art of Birth group, we are able to develop a supportive relationship with the facilitator and other group members).

Through the therapeutic benefits of art we can generate self-esteem, gain confidence and empower ourselves to be more in control of our life. The creative process can enhance emotional well-being in absolutely anyone who is willing to try it. All of our desires and all of our answers lie within us, so give yourself permission to go on a journey within – at any time – and see for yourself what may emerge out of your creations.

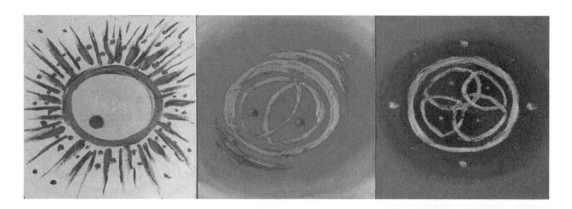

In The Beginning 1, 2, 3 – paintings by Alexandra Florschutz

There are many cultures who believe what happens in the womb during pregnancy is a microcosmic reflection of the universe. There is also a belief that art is a reflection of the soul and it relates to the heart, not the intellect. According to Steiner, painting is controlled by the Ego (higher self) and is a breathing process which opens the heart. Birth must be approached from the heart, not the head, and although giving birth is an effort of the Will, thoughts that are positive are very helpful. We can, therefore, heal our fear-based thoughts and feelings through artistic expression, connecting to the heart at the same time. It is a process of surrendering intellectual self control and hand over the power to our body and allow it to do its job. It is often the mind that stands in the way of us being able to fully 'let go' of being in control or making a mess. Birth is messy and art is often a messy experience! Preparation of the mind can support this letting go as there is nothing left for the mind to hold on to if the emotional way is clear. Making art that is messy or seems to be out of control also helps us to relinquish our self control and revel in freedom. Therefore, art can help us enter this primal state more quickly and tune into the wisdom of the body in preparation for birth.

Steiner expanded on the arts and explains how they are connected to the elements: 'Warmth rules in the air, musically; Air (with its attendant light conditions) rules in the water, pictorially; and water rules in the earth (or solidity) sculpturally' (Houschka-Stavenhagen, M. 2005, p62). Perhaps this concept is something to mull over rather than to analyse its meaning straight away.

'The arts cease to be merely the specialised domains of talented persons. They become once more a possession of all humanity – each one of them is so, when one understands them in their connection with human nature' (Houschka-Stavenhagen, M. 2005, p70).

When looked at in this way, our artistic expression is our birth right; it is for everyone! The creative arts are the fundamental principle of existence.

Creating space for yourself to be creative and explore how it feels to be pregnant is both soothing and potentially enlightening.

Art has the power to access unconscious processes which can find an outlet for healing or venting by making them conscious. The very nature of creativity complements the creative process of pregnancy and is therefore the most compatible form of self exploration.

✦ Art is a way of knowing what we actually believe (Pat B. Allen)

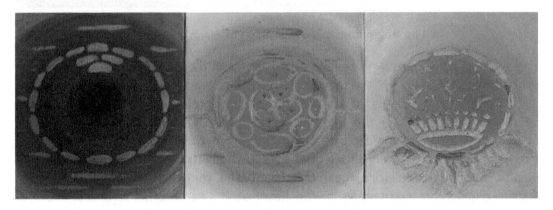

In The Beginning 4, 5, 6 – paintings by Alexandra Florschutz

All children have the ability to draw/scribble/paint; it is only life and situations, like school (which emphasises technical skill, intellectual approach and good grades), that interrupt this most natural form of expression. Dr Winnicott talks about the importance of being creative and the ability to play in order to maintain a healthy sense of self. If adults are unable to use art or be creative, it is not because art is not for ALL; it is because they have been hindered in some form during their life. When people engage with art materials, the outcome is often very liberating.

'... The expression of unconscious wishes and feelings, even in disguised form in a drawing, serves as a "safety valve" which provides a harmless discharge of feelings which would otherwise be "bottled up" and possibly dangerous... drawing may allow the catharsis (purging) of repressed emotions... and the suggestion... that play provides an opportunity for the harmless expression of instinctive impulses'. (Thomas, G. V., & Silk, A. M. J. 1989).

Nora Swan-Foster, an art therapist who works with pregnant women in the US, believes that 'the active art process best suits a pregnant woman because it offers a sublimated way to experience prenatal bonding, separation through childbirth and post partum bonding... Thus, the personal imagery is used to increase self-awareness rather than remaining as unresolved anxiety that may interrupt the mother/child relationship'. It is possible 'also to actively mobilize the vivid imagery to transform the fears and conflicts into new imagery that empowers the woman as a mother' (Swan-Foster, N. 1989).

Joan Raphael-Leff, a psychotherapist working with pregnant women worldwide, suggests that prenatal therapy can help reduce 'the likelihood of postnatal depression and suicidal attempts, possibly preventing obstetric complications, and pre-empting the long-term effects of pathological parent-baby interactions, child abuse, and emotional neglect' (Raphael-Leff 1995)!

If this kind of emotional support was offered by the National Health Service in mainstream hospitals, as a routine service for pregnant women, then we might begin to see improved ante natal and post natal outcomes. Birth with less obstetric complications/interventions would not only be more cost effective but, more importantly, would benefit pregnant women. Reducing psychological barriers to the birth process is paramount. Positive and anxiety-reducing interventions during pregnancy are likely to promote better engagement by women in ante natal care, which would greatly increase the chance of good birth and post natal outcomes such as higher chance of breast feeding and better child health. A creative programme has the potential to reduce psychological morbidity associated with pregnancy, birth and the postnatal period.

Pregnancy and art transcend class and culture and can change lives as well as change childbirth. Let us be the catalyst for positive change.

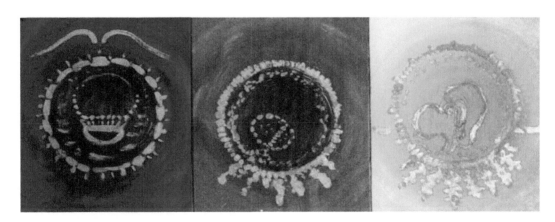

In The Beginning 7, 8, 9 – paintings by Alexandra Florschutz

A Brief History of Art Therapy

In the late 1940's, artist Adrian Hill was recovering from tuberculosis. He experimented with art materials and discovered the therapeutic benefits of art – because 'it completely engrosses the mind as well as the fingers and releases the creative energy of the frequently inhibited patient' which, he suggested, 'enabled the patient to build up a strong defence against his misfortunes' (Hill, 1948, p103). Although pregnant women are not patients, Hill offers an interesting example of how the use of art helped him recover from illness.

Around the same time Margaret Naumberg – a Psychologist in the USA – began to use art in her therapy work and went on to call it art therapy. One could say Margaret Naumberg promoted the use of art in therapy while Adrian Hill advocated art as therapy.

Art Therapy developed along two parallel strands - Art as therapy and art psychotherapy. One emphasises the 'healing' potential of art, whereas the second stresses the importance of the therapeutic relationship established between the art therapist, the client and the artwork (usually with a psychodynamic approach). This is often referred to as the triangular relationship. Nowadays art therapy is recognised as a synthesis between the two and although many professions use art as a tool, art therapy is a profession practiced by highly trained art therapists or art psychotherapists.

The Art of Feminine Sexuality

What is it to be a Woman in our time? What does the Feminine actually mean? What is the definition of Feminine Power? I am on a journey exploring what may be the Source of a woman's power, the feminine spirit which thrived in the more female oriented Goddess cultures, only to be superseded by the patriarchal way of life. I wonder how we can retain the true nature of our gender while navigating this predominantly masculine driven world – what does life look like from the Feminine point of view? When I say 'masculine', I mean it in the broader sense which refers to the masculine principle: physical, active, linear, driven, goal oriented, achieving, independent, money, external and not necessarily 'male'. The feminine principle has been described as the contrast or opposite: internal, unconscious, intuitive, round, feeling, night, moon, receptive and more flowing. Many women tend to approach life, nowadays, from the more masculine perspective, as a result of our culture and how we are raised. Schools only focus on educating the intellect with constant testing so we reach our intended goal which is to pass the exam in the expected format. The fight for gender equality has resulted in women simulating the masculine model, without developing our feminine power as an equal. This has created the tendency to become like a 'superwoman', juggling careers, family and social lives which inevitably leaves us exhausted at the end of the day. This can often be in conflict with our deeper dreams and desires in life and especially when it comes to the process of pregnancy and birth which requires the more intuitive body wisdom and knowledge. I have been on an exciting journey of self discovery and my passionate insights into feminine sexuality aim to unlock a whole other dimension in the wonderful domain of being a woman.

'Aspects of female sexuality include issues pertaining to biological sex, body image, self-esteem, personality, sexual orientation, values, attitudes, gender roles, relationships, activity options, and communication' (http://en.wikipedia.org/wiki/Human_female_sexuality). Interestingly it does not mention birth which is the most momentous event a woman can experience in her body/genitalia, mind and spirit!

My personal art work, as an artist, explores the themes of conception, birth, feminine sexuality and how this can be represented in the cycles of nature and life. Visit www.florschutz.com.

My desire for women to become integrated in self knowledge, acceptance and love is paramount. This integration can happen when we live in choice, respecting our body and mind and avoid handing over our dreams to the constriction of accepted social mores.

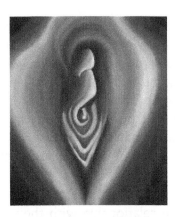

Divine Source, Shell – painting by Alexandra Florschutz

When it comes to the female genitalia, there are so many words for the different parts which can sometimes cause confusion. The word vagina is often misused because it refers specifically to an interior structure, whereas the Vulva is the whole exterior genitalia. The vulva has many major and minor anatomical components, including the mons pubis, labia majora, labia minora, clitoris, bulb of vestibule, vulval vestibule, greater and lesser vestibular glands, and the opening of the vagina. The vagina is like the bridge between the external vulva genitalia and the magical internal system of cervix, fallopian tubes, ovaries and uterus. The clitoris, a little ball-like organ, is situated above the opening of the urethra and is purely designed for sexual pleasure. Eight thousand nerve endings (twice as many as the male penis) culminate in the clitoris which is all connected to the vulva, vagina and the rest of the body. The clitoris, or 'pleasure central', allows orgasm without penetration. Orgasms release powerful health giving endorphins/dopamine, the chemicals of well-being and have often been associated with enhancing a woman's creativity. It is not surprising then that some cultures, who wish to suppress female power and retain docile obedience, surgically remove the clitoris!

The female reproductive system and genitalia are the most impressive parts of being a woman and yet they have been the most shamed, abused and violated. Women have become sexualised objects, where external features define a woman as 'good enough' for the male gaze and any natural bodily functions are suppressed or extensively sanitised. The vagina, in particular, is still seen as shameful, dirty or 'looks wrong' and the expectation is that only a man can ignite its pleasure. Even language has encouraged negative connotations: vagina is the general anatomical term which suggests 'clinical detachment' (Camphausen, R. C. 1996), vulva is a bit vague, and the word cunt (which, like vulva, means female external genital organs), is the most insulting word used today but has derived from the Greek fertility goddess Kunthus and the Indian nature/earth goddess Kunti (I'm sure amongst other positive derivatives). In the Middle Ages, the word cunt was the everyday factual word used in England instead of vagina or vulva which was brought over by the Anglo-Saxons. It was also normal, during this period, for streets to be named after the trade that took place there and so a red light district became known as Gropecunt Lane. Gradually the word became associated with prostitution and as women and their sexuality, as a source of power, were feared by men, it is not surprising that cunt has become a derogatory expletive. Thankfully the Sanskrit word Yoni translates as Womb, Origin, Source and Vulva and is somewhat more appropriate in my opinion, albeit borrowed from an ancient culture. I, however, like to refer to the Yoni as a woman's Divine Source © because it is the gateway to physical pleasure and the creation of new life which collectively embodies her entire life energy.

As women cultivate a positive relationship with their divine source, they discover the power of their intuitive compass as a way to navigate life. I want to raise awareness and show how unique, beautiful and sacred your divine source is and release the man-made guilt and shame that has been attached to our most precious anatomical gem for centuries. I think the divine source is the symbol of the feminine spirit and where a woman holds her natural power. The anatomical genitalia are only the external expression of a complex internal system of pleasure, reproduction and for the creation of new life. This system embraces the three lower Chakras; the root, the sacral and the solar plexus and their primary function is sexuality, reproduction and energy. This is the centre of a woman's powerful creative force which ultimately generates her life energy.

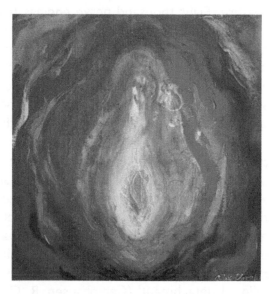

Divine Source, Fire – painting by Alexandra Florschutz

If we relate to our sexuality or genitalia with guilt, shame, disgust or anger, then how is this going to affect our overall self esteem and the generally messy, physical, earthiness of giving birth? We all started life inside a woman's body and entered the world, in most cases, via her genitalia. As more than half of all births require medical intervention and many are very traumatic I think this stresses the importance for a change in attitude to our genitalia and how we use our energy. I believe birth is another covert way by which the predominantly masculine medical profession (aka the patriarchy, which can include women) controls, violates and abuses a woman's body when she gives birth. The message is that a woman cannot give birth without the assistance of technology, drugs or surgery. Birth is the most natural thing in the world and the most powerful rite of passage we as women can experience, but most of us have lost our intuitive inner compass which allows us to know exactly what to do and when to do it. We need to get into agreement with our body; it is perfect, innocent, beautiful and life-giving. We must take back the baton of self-love and refrain from making pregnancy and birth a total inconvenience. We must also stop pursuing outer physical perfection, or to satisfy people's expectations, our primary goal. Pleasure is our birth right not our shame. The more we build a relationship with our body and listen to its messages, the easier it will be to self care, know our deepest desires, love and respect ourselves and open up to the act of giving birth. Let us reclaim our sacred sexuality before birth. I like to use the stunning Lotus flower as a symbol of utter innocence, beauty, sacred sexuality and openness. If we cultivate the qualities of our inner world, such as Imagination, Inspiration and Intuition – a co creative process of mind AND heart which is our divine right and attainable by personal exploration – then I believe women will truly change the world!

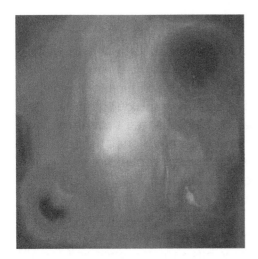

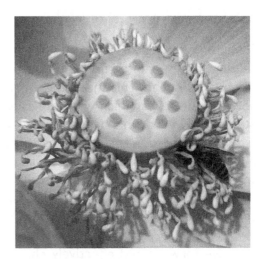

Intimacy – painting   **Pink Lotus with Bee** – photograph
both by Alexandra Florschutz

From Feminism to Feminine Power – A New Perspective

There appears to be two dimensions to being a woman in the 21st Century. The first seems to be the increasing competition between the sexes, particularly in the Western world. Women have taken on the masculine power system and although we have levelled the so called playing field, studies have shown that women are much less happy than they used to be despite the apparent equality. Women are lead to believe that to be accepted and taken seriously in the world or the workplace they have to be as capable, successful (both financially and professionally) and as strong as men. Working women enter the business arena of men, set up by men to suit their way of operating. This is fine for men but women often work in a different way, or would work in a different way given half a chance. If women also want to have children then it usually becomes an either or situation or a stressful combination. Women go to work and have to pretend they do not have children. The glass ceiling syndrome still seems to exist which is reflected in the current statistic of around 8% of women CEOs worldwide in 2012, which is appalling. If there was a valued 'Feminine way' of working then women could become successful without having to simulate the masculine way of the workplace unless they really wanted to work within that model. (http://en.wikipedia.org/wiki/List_of_female_top_executives)

Feminism, although it began with the Suffragettes in the late 19th and early 20th century, finally erupted in the 1960's with anger; anger at men, the patriarchy, and the establishment. This made the world wake up to the global unjust inequalities between the sexes which was desperately needed and my gratitude to my sisters is eternal. However, on a deeper level, not a great deal has changed since then as we are still fighting our corner, trying to gain supremacy. Anger is still at the heart of our struggle to equalise the sexes and gain respect and power. Although anger is an instinctive response to unfairness or inequality and can be the catalyst for change, it is not necessarily the overall solution. The injustice that provokes the anger is the problem – a social problem. How can we positively channel our anger towards all the flagitious crimes that are committed against women daily in order to move forward and effectively change this atrocious situation once and for all? Despite the valiant efforts to tackle gender-based violence by organisations like the World Health Organisation (WHO), the statistics show that violence towards women is on the increase!

'The United Nations defines violence against women as "any act of gender-based violence that results in, or is likely to result in, physical, sexual or mental harm or suffering to women, including threats of such acts, coercion or arbitrary deprivation of liberty, whether occurring in public or in private life'.

'A WHO multi-country study found that between 15-71% of women aged 15-49 years reported physical and/or sexual violence by an intimate partner at some point in their lives' (information taken from WHO website dated November 2012). http://www.who.int/mediacentre/factsheets/fs239/en/.

The Ministry of Justice, Home Office and the Office for National Statistics UK and Wales Report for 2011/2012, states that 'around one in twenty females (aged 16 to 59) reported being a victim of a most serious sexual offence since the age of 16. Extending this to include other sexual offences such as sexual threats, unwanted touching or indecent exposure, this increased to one in five females reporting being a victim since the age of 16'. It also shows that 20% of women experienced sexual abuse as children.http://www.justice.gov.uk/statistics/criminal-justice/sexual-offending-statistics

These statistics show that it is almost impossible for women NOT to be in a perpetual state of angry uproar. On the one hand these top organisations continue to campaign for gender equality and yet crimes against women appear to be escalating. Why is this? It suggests that as women strive towards and achieve autonomy, the men are fighting back to gain control. It brings us back to the psychological tenet, that if we blame a person, the very act of being blamed causes a defence which creates a desire to fight back. Women are fighting for their rights, men feel blamed and so fight back to prove their perceived innocence which perpetuates a vicious circle. It is thought that if we do not fight our cause then 'they' win. We could say that it is a war worth fighting but as we know, war only fuels war. How can we continue our campaign in a more peaceful way and achieve permanent change?

I believe that if as many women as possible in the world can become peaceful activists, then we can set an example for the rest of the world. If we take responsibility for our choices and actions and not project all the blame onto men or the patriarchy, then this might help to move us forward. By generating a shift in consciousness we could create a new dialogue between the sexes. I also think we can make faster progress if we recruit the more enlightened men on our side and co create change together.

⚜ Nothing ever goes away until it teaches us what we need to know (Pema Chodron)

To take this one step further, I think the dark forces of materialism currently sweeping the globe, including the technological take over, are accentuating the existing patriarchal paradigm. Materialism encourages our reliance on technology, undermines all that is natural, common sense, intuitive, or self aware and makes us dependent on the system. We can see how this is translated in art, architecture, materials, media and the perpetuation of violence particularly prevalent in Play Station/Xbox games. These games are mainly targeted at younger boys who are seduced by the macho, power hungry, violent, fake male role models who perform gratuitous violence and objectify women. The brainwashing of our impressionable children by normalising violence and war for boys and over sexualising our young girls causing permanent body image dissatisfaction, will require a new wave of brave parents to raise conscious, creative children who can lead the world towards positive change and a new way of being.

Feminism seems to assume that the Feminine is less powerful than the masculine. I think that feminism can sometimes undermine the Feminine and being a woman at times. We need to stand strong in our feminine principle, as there is masculine and feminine everywhere in nature and in ourselves. We are equal and yet totally different. The Feminine is as powerful and we can only find balance if we also embrace the masculine. It is interesting to note the meaning of the word 'power' in the dictionary which describes it as the ability to *do* something (it is active); political, financial or social authority; authority of a person or group; a position of control. This is quite characteristic of the masculine principle (which is fine) while women tend to want inclusivity, connection, support, and to effect positive change and not necessarily have control or power over people for personal triumph. We still want to be valued for our contribution and women usually desire power so they can positively transform the system. So for want of a better word, feminine power must find its natural expression in the world and not shy away from feeling inadequate or lash out in defensiveness. Men love seeing women thrive in their feminine power but not in competition with their own way of operating. I believe we will be more powerful by honouring the Feminine principle than by fighting the 'other'.

On the one hand, western women have choices but on the other hand, women in some parts of the world are still controlled, abused, denied an education, considered second class citizens, or even murdered because they are a girl, or because they speak out, or are gay, or they dare to break free. While the two extremes exist and this gap is possibly widening, there is still a central domain where women are searching for a new meaning of the Feminine.

> **Because women are often caged early on in life by the culture, the over culture has expectations that the radiance and enormity of the Feminine should somehow be squished or squashed down and condensed into a much smaller version (Clarissa Pinkola Estes, Seeing in the Dark CD, Side 1).**

Women in the West are privileged to have such freedom that women in other cultures do not possess. In the West, I believe we will never feel valued or 'equal' to men unless we feel it in the depth of our being! Equality begins at home and by that I mean within each and every woman. We do not have to have a high powered job to feel equal because the chances are that, if we do not feel equal within ourselves, or value our uniqueness, then the outside world will reflect this back to us by undermining our performance, or ideas, even if we are in the highest paid and respected job. This so called equality is really self-love and self-approval. Women in other cultures do not have this luxury. It is time for us to Choose how we live and work from the 'Feminine' perspective, enjoy being Women and release the competitive drive against men that becomes so exhausting. Let us leave Superwoman in the Comics where she belongs because we are totally good enough, beautiful and lovable exactly the way we are Now! Let us set men free to go on their journey and allow them the honour of supporting us (in all forms not necessarily financial) and not feel undermined by their service towards the Feminine. I think women will become more powerful in the world, in business, in our financial rewards, in raising children and so on, if we begin to promote and design our careers and families working from the Feminine perspective. It really comes down to valuing our uniqueness and not looking outside our selves for approval from men or society.

We can also play with the notion of the masculine and feminine principles within our own psyches. In simplistic terms, the feminine part of our being has the idea and the masculine puts it into action. They both work together! We could also say, what is without, is also within and by that I mean balancing the masculine and feminine principles in the world and also within our Selves to create an existence where men and women complement each other – not compete for power.

⊥ If you could trust your dreams half as much as you doubt them, you would get everything you want (Regena Thomashauer, a.k.a. Mama Gena)

We must also remember that Women are ruled by cycles with our main one being connected to the moon. When girls reach puberty and they start their menses, the whole show begins. Every month she will experience a change, maybe feel more fragile or introspective (and every woman's experience is different). In older cultures women used to congregate together and menstruate or give birth supported by each other. Nowadays menstruation is seen as a total inconvenience, especially in the work place where we are supposed to be super efficient, switched on, focussed and goal oriented. There is also big business around 'feminine hygiene', suggesting we are 'dirty' during this time. We are not allowed to smell, have hair, be slightly overweight, or anything that would deem us less than perfect. The media consistently projects the message that women are only acceptable if they look, act, or are a certain way that suits the male gaze – and now this message is being projected by women, to women, as well! Once again, we choose the way in which we wish to respond to these messages.

Then our sexual desires awaken in adolescence and we are caught in a confusing contradiction of double standards where boys are patted on the back for having sex or losing their virginity while girls are called derogatory names if they do the same. The message is that it is ok for men to be sexual while women are supposed to be 'pure', and yet they are expected to engage sexually or be called frigid or a tease. I know this is a clichéd generalised picture but the underlying message still prevails. Advertising also promotes the perfect sexy pubescent girl who is ripe and ready to seduce every man into bed. But in reality, girls have always been told to behave like ladies, not to touch their 'down there' region, not to show their knickers, not be provocative and be 'good girls' and suppress their natural, vibrant sexuality. Then teenage girls feel they have to simulate the advertising image of a 'good enough' woman by presenting themselves in a sexually provocative way in order to be noticed by the opposite sex. I think this is ludicrous! Why can't girls be given permission to grow up knowing that their sexuality is innocent, sacred and something they are in charge of and that self pleasuring is normal and healthy. And that they should never rely on the opposite sex to validate their fabulousness. If they desire a sexual encounter with a guy, then it is their choice or desire and not because they feel they 'should' consent for fear of ridicule. Another common situation is that women think they will receive love and acceptance if they engage sexually with a man (i.e. give sex to receive love). Sex should be for their pleasure only or at least mutual pleasure and intimacy and not only to please a man. Developing intimacy with another human being leads to greater sexual pleasure than promiscuity which may seem more exciting at the time but does not lead to fulfilment in the long run.

Women are the mothers of humanity and they nurture the consciousness of society in their wombs (Dansby, B. A. 2000)

Women are the birth keepers! We are responsible for bearing the next generation of this planet – with a man's help of course! Birth is a wonderful aspect of being a woman (if we choose to have children) – the gift to give birth. We menstruate to cleanse the womb for potential pregnancies. Pregnancy is often a rocky road for women and birth is usually approached with a sense of resignation that it is going to be difficult. How can we give birth naturally – which is a real joy when that happens – when the medical profession still controls this event and postulate the message that birth should be in hospital under the direction of nurses and doctors. Once again, if we trust our body and have the integrated experience that our sexuality is normal, safe, sacred and innocent (i.e. the opposite to guilt and shame which is still present) then we can approach birth from a more positive perspective.

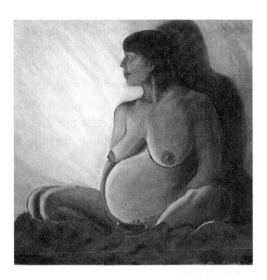

Waiting (Pregnant Woman) – painting by Alexandra Florschutz

Menopause, the next cycle of being a woman, is a stage from which we can emerge as powerful and radiant, sexual goddesses. We leave our child bearing ability behind us, and enter a freer, wiser phase of powerful creative potential. However, according to society and the media, we are not allowed to be 'old'! Again, we need to take back our power and rejoice being a mature woman. If we 'approve' of our self, then the world will follow. It all starts with the individual. Let us live from the Wild Woman sentiment, follow our dreams and love our precious selves first and foremost!

How are we going to 'educate' or 'empower' women to love and approve of themselves, in the West and in poorer countries? How are we going to set an example, so we become positive beacons worthy of following? We do not want to give the message that the only way to be a 'real woman' is to hand over our power and compete for recognition or validation by the patriarchal system. If we wish to empower Women of the world to have self respect and self approval then we must develop that first and be the example!

♣ You must be the change you wish to see in the world (Gandhi)

We can learn a great deal of positive attributes, skills and traits from men, the masculine and patriarchy. We now realise that we can have a lucrative career or be entrepreneurs and pay our way. We know how to negotiate the best energy tariff, we can find the most suitable mortgage or car insurance, vote, be company directors, run our own business and we can have children on our own! Men offer their own unique perspective on life and create an all needed balance. Even though the female evolution is still being undermined, it is perhaps time we reinterpret the fight and redefine the status quo.

We can certainly pay homage to our wonderful courageous Sisters who have pioneered for the past 100 years to wake the world up to women's inequality and yet in this age of desired peace, we need to evolve towards a positive paradigm to move us forward. It is now about empowering, educating, honouring and loving ourselves first and not looking at men for the answers, the permission, the approval or for *them* to be the ones to exert change. Let us join forces and stand united in our quest. Let us awaken the Feminine for the new age and celebrate ourselves as being fabulous women!

I think it is about transforming the goddess culture and the current god culture which is clearly on the way out, and moving forward in self knowledge and wisdom. It doesn't need to be a battle anymore in the West – we are our own authority and no man (or woman) can say otherwise. Our spirit is equal and free and resides along the spectrum in the realm of the Feminine, next to the wonderful Masculine.

If we aim to be the change we want to see in the world, as Ghandi said, then let us positively develop our own Feminine potential – which I think is a balance between the inner masculine and feminine principles – and leave men to sort out their own perspective. If we deny one principle, then the balance shifts to one sidedness. Women are over developing the masculine and more often than not squashing the Feminine because we subconsciously believe it is less effective or weak! I think both genders need to aim towards being whole and complete.

⚜ Creativity will balance out the prevalent intellectual one-sidedness of our materialistic culture. We need the Arts now more than ever

I believe the role of the new Feminist is about Acquired Wisdom not a competitive gender war. We somehow have to lead the way in the business/corporate world, not by simulating the masculine model – as we are currently doing – but by leading the way from the Feminine perspective even if we borrow so called masculine attributes. For example, I know of many campaigns to reduce pornography, prostitution, to abolish topless pictures in newspapers (i.e. Page 3 in the British Newspaper The Sun) and other outrageous reductions of a woman's self worth but it still takes a woman to consent to such actions (if they are not coerced or abducted into this business). Perhaps a woman would not enter into such an industry if she valued her Self but she is also entitled to do so if she desires to take that path (and I am not talking about the manipulation of vulnerable women who are driven by poverty and ignorant to lucrative offers that turn out to be false). The world is going through immense change and it is now crucial that we stand united in the Feminine model. What this means exactly, is still up for discussion but I do think it has a lot to do with self worth and taking care of our needs but in the meantime we can work towards gaining deeper clarity. If we hold that thought, then it will be a good starting point.

One fundamental element within this renewed Feminine Principle is a time to honour our children once more. This is NOT done by returning to the passive mother role of bygone years 'chained to the kitchen sink' but re-learning to enjoy our children and see the role of the parent as being the most important job in the world. I think a more balanced approach does exist in European countries like Denmark where the role of the father is highly valued. We must end the perpetual cycle of passing down our issues to our children and creating the next generation of wounded adults who then go on to educate their own children in the same modality. Children are such wonderful beings and can be our greatest teachers. Sadly, in the UK, women are increasingly defined by their 'job'. The government promotes going back to work and makes it possible for women to do that as soon as they can by offering financial assistance towards childcare instead of supporting the mother (or father) to look after their own children if they desire. This message is so powerful that it is not acceptable to be 'a stay at home mum' anymore and I hear comments everyday 'I'm just a mum'! I am, however, in total support of both camps. I think women have a divine right to work in whatever career they desire – to follow their bliss – AND have a right to look after their own children. There needs to be a shift in consciousness that, first, values the role of motherhood (and fatherhood) and as a result given more emotional and financial support. Second, makes the workplace more supportive to women who have children that need or want to work. It comes down to making choices out of a sense of freedom not from underlying 'should' feelings of guilt.

I have included a list of the group of archetypal Greek goddesses who embody particular timeless characteristics which I think are synonymous with contemporary women. I think it gives a wonderful example of how diverse a woman's qualities are and that although we talk about the Feminine principle, it does not mean all women have to be the same. I have always been more of an Aphrodite, Demeter and Persephone woman but in more recent years have developed Artemis and Hestia traits. I am still working on my Hera attributes! We can all identify with one or more of these Goddessly qualities and this will also have a bearing on the way we approach birth. Maybe the archetypal Feminine is an integration of all the goddess characters?

⚓ Women have an all knowing medial nature, which we can rekindle at any time

Artemis (Diana) – Goddess of the hunt and moon. She is independent, focussed on her target which she is able to reach with clarity. She is autonomous and self sufficient.

Athena (Minerva) – Goddess of wisdom and crafts. She is an alpha female who is intellectual, career oriented, good at problem solving, and embodies much of the masculine characteristics.

Hestia (Vesta) – Goddess of the hearth and temple. She is more comfortable creating her beautiful home and likes her own company. She is also inclined to be more spiritual.

Hera (Juno) – Goddess of marriage. She is a devoted wife and values marriage and fidelity.

Demeter (Ceres) – Goddess of the grain. She is the ultimate earth mother, maternal in all ways, abundant, caring and generous.

Persephone (Proserpina) – Goddess maiden and queen of the underworld. Creative, receptive, has a developed relationship with the unconscious dream world of imagination and intuition.

Aphrodite (Venus) – Goddess of love and beauty. She is an alchemical goddess who enjoys being creative, sensual and loves all things pleasurable and beautiful.

The Pink Tent Art Installation

The Pink Tent is an Art Installation I created to celebrate the Feminine and initiate dialogue. It has appeared in many venues such as art exhibitions, festivals, women's gatherings, health and wellbeing fairs, to inspire women and men to ask the question: what does it mean to be a woman in our (Western) culture? It offers a safe space for discussion on this huge topic. It is a celebration of all things feminine. It allows women to expand their self awareness of who they are beyond the context of our culture while giving a positive insight for men. A place where people can have a creative, sensual, informative and transformative felt experience of the Feminine – a space to co-create this notion.

The Pink Tent contains themes such as: female cycles, pregnancy and birth, feminine sexuality, menopause, the different aspects of the Goddess, the pursuit of our own pleasure, inner acceptance and happiness.

The Goddesses, which can be described as female archetypes, conjure different characteristics such as strength, love, home, freedom, peace, sensuality, etc. The goddess is also about 'Birth, Growth, Death and Regeneration' (M. Gimbutas).

Pink is symbolic of love, beauty, femininity, compassion, motherhood, emotional and spiritual healing and much more and is a combination of Red (earth, passion) and White (purity and contains all colours). Pink is a higher vibration to red and is connected to the heart chakra.

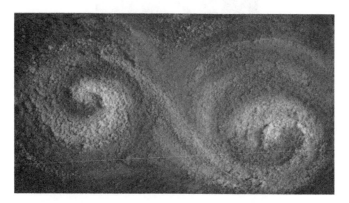

Pink Spiral – painting by Alexandra Florschutz

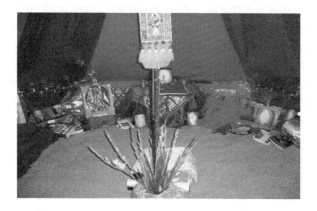

The Pink Tent Art Installation (interior)

In 2012, I supported a V-Day event at Sussex University in the UK where they organised a week of interesting talks, workshops and films culminating with a performance of Eve Ensler's The Vagina Monologues. I put my Tent up in the centre of the campus during their 'Wellness Fair' and spent the whole day talking to many people, the majority female, about their experience of being a woman. The consistent response was quite shocking to me and I realised that the whole Feminist movement had not really changed very much in the way women perceive themselves in relationship to men. One must bear in mind that the general age range was early twenties which is the newer generation compared to my own generation. They were following the same courses as men which suggests welcome educational equality. They did, however, express the ongoing culture of sexism towards women and that they did not feel safe as women (the highest occurrence of rape is during university years). Motherhood was not regarded as a worthwhile way to spend your life and they still did not feel like equals to their masculine peers.

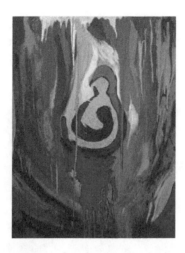

Mother & Child – painting by Alexandra Florschutz

What is going on?

In one way, there is now a natural progression for boys and girls to be educated in the same way, studying the same subjects, going to college or university (or getting a job), to finding an appropriate career so their independent life can be financially covered. There is nothing wrong with any of that but the current establishment does not offer any education about the uniqueness of being a woman, so women can feel understood and men can appreciate them because they have received a positive picture of what it means to be a woman.

The masculine is independent while the feminine works well in groups, they need connection (we all do). Women need to cultivate independence within themselves while we allow the 'group' of women to support us. We do not need to battle it alone. We can lovingly hold each other accountable to walk our talk and follow our bliss. Love, praise, build each other up, not judge, undermine, or be one up on each other. We do not need to rely on men to validate this for us, as they have no understanding what it is to be a woman, so it takes the pressure off them and leaves us freer to enjoy our relationships with men in a more healthy way.

This is a really positive time to redefine our current paradigm. Luckily there are many groups emerging, with many wonderful women who carry the torch towards this change. Let us support these initiatives wholeheartedly so our message can spread in a healthy way and continue the Feminist work in peace, love and joy.

⬥ **Women must not feel that they all have to be the same in order to qualify to be part of the Feminine camp!**

A Potential Solution

This brings me to one potential solution which I believe overrides anything I have said previously and that is the wonderful world of Pleasure! If we find our own pleasure in all we do, whether it is taking a walk in the woods, drinking tea from our best china, picking a beautiful rose just for our own enjoyment, deciding to have a dance break when we feel like the gloom is coming to get us, or having fun no matter how mundane we think something is, then we never have to rely on external factors to give it to us. Pleasure can lead the way to our fulfilled dreams. We certainly cannot be a martyr if we follow our pleasure! If we truly want to be powerful women in any of our choices whether this is being a parent, a career woman, or both, then we MUST learn to look after our own needs, desires and pleasures. This does NOT mean that we will not be supported, looked after, pampered or treated like a goddess but we have to know what we want first and learn the art of asking for it in a way that is pleasurable to both ourselves and others.

⬧ **Pleasure increases Oxytocin which reduces stress (Dr John Gray)**

One way of tuning into our pleasure is through our creativity. Re-connecting to our creativity through Art can fast track us to our pleasure. I certainly find painting an aphrodisiac which is good news when it comes to pregnancy and birth because a relaxed cervix delivers a baby more easily and with increased pleasure. Experiencing our body's sensual pleasure is not only grounding but takes us out of our heads which is so necessary when birthing and is aligned to the way it all started – making love! Let us make birth a pleasurable experience and harness the power of our creative forces to birth our babies and our projects with the juicy, sublime pleasure that is available to us all.

Regina Thomashauer, a.k.a. Mama Gena, started the School of Womanly Arts to explore the lost art of enjoying our life through pleasure. She describes her teaching as 'identifying your desires, having fun no matter where you are, knowing sensual pleasure, befriending your inner bitch, flirting (in a way that makes your day, not just his), and more – because making pleasure your priority can actually help you reach your goals.' There is a lot of truth in what she talks about which often gets bypassed on our self development path because of our fast track desire for spiritual enlightenment. We often forget to enjoy our life in this moment and remember that we can actually be the catalyst to making our moment enjoyable, fun and even ecstatic. What can you do for yourself today that brings you pleasure?

I have been committed to leading a pleasurable life for some time now and am always being mindful of living from this place of fulfilment (whenever possible). I believe pleasure is the key to one's liberation and it empowers a woman/the Feminine. Also, pleasure is multi layered and personal (what works for me may not pleasure you), so I enjoy my own personal pleasure research in every moment. My list is endless! What does your list look like?

🔸 **Pleasure comes from giving yourself permission to explore your appetites freely, with no guilt (R. Thomashauer, 2002. *Mama Gena's School of Womanly Arts*).**

Ecstatic Birth

'The way a woman gives birth is intimately intertwined with her approach to life and sensuality. Ecstatic Birth is a call to reconfigure our cultural conception of birth. It is a call to put childbirth back on its sacred pedestal and women back into an empowered relationship with their bodies and their experience of birth' (Sheila Kamara Hay www.ecstatic-birth.com). I think this says it all.

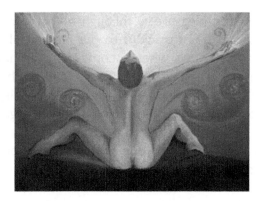

Ecstatic Feminine – Painting by Alexandra Florschutz

My Art

My artwork explores themes such as pregnancy, birth, feminine sexuality and being a woman. I have developed a variety of symbolic ways of representing these themes in addition to more realistic or representational work.

The Spiral is a circle set free. It stands for the ancient symbol of the goddess, the womb, fertility, feminine serpent force, continual change, and the evolution of the universe. It is also associated with the solar calendar, the rhythm of the seasons and the cycle of birth, death and rebirth. The Lotus Flower symbolises purity, the ultimate feminine sexuality and divine birth. I represent the Divine Source as a symbol of creative feminine power.

The Divine Source© series represents the symbol of the feminine spirit and where a woman holds her natural power. The anatomical genitalia are only the external expression of a complex internal system of pleasure, reproduction and for the creation of new life.

The technique I use begins with a particular evocative colour mood and the nascent image evolves out of this colour infusion. My paintings often combine a variety of tactile media which is not only a pleasurable experience but allows the viewer to enter into a world of deep colour, sparkles and magic.

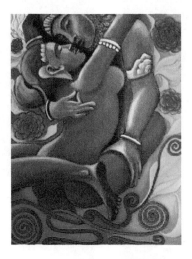 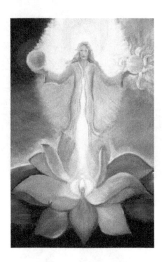

Lovers　　　　　　　　　　**Goddess Sophia**

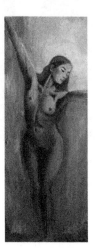 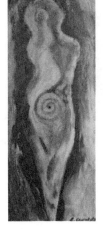

Divine Source Goddess 1 & 2

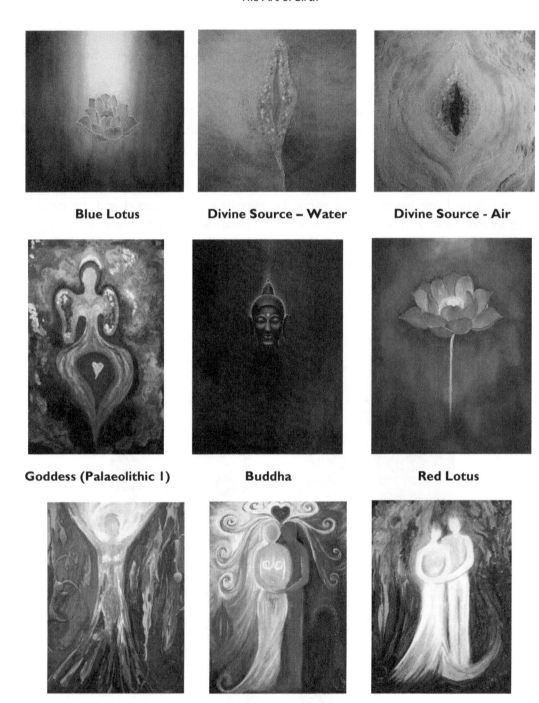

Blue Lotus   **Divine Source – Water**   **Divine Source - Air**

Goddess (Palaeolithic 1)   **Buddha**   **Red Lotus**

Passionate Feminine   **Sacred Union**   **Fairy Lovers**

A Sensitive Subject

Healing Pregnancy Loss – Miscarriage

It is important to mention pregnancy loss because it affects many women and their partners. Pregnancy loss can include, 'failed in vitro fertilization, molar pregnancy, ectopic pregnancy, loss in multiple-gestation pregnancy, abortion, miscarriage and stillbirth' (Seftel L., 2006). Couples express that they do not always know how to grieve because they are not sure if they have lost a group of cells, a foetus or a child. Some families find it helpful to give their baby foetus a burial, choose a name, and grieve the gap that is left in the family unit. I hear women say 'I have three children but only two living'. Some women remain in denial about how they feel about their miscarriage until they are given permission to unlock their emotions. A woman may feel there is something wrong with their body, there may also be guilt if she feels relieved and a myriad of emotions that are unique to her experience. All feelings are the truth for the individual. Nevertheless, you may be filled with a void that you are not sure how to express. I think whatever your feelings are they need to be validated, expressed and grieved as you wish, knowing that you are completely entitled to all your feelings. Society does not really talk about this subject or give it importance unless you have direct experience. It is really helpful to acknowledge your feelings, if you haven't already, especially before your next pregnancy or birth.

Miscarriage is very common and can cause anxiety in subsequent pregnancies. It may trigger feelings of physical and emotional loss but women and families do not receive the support they deserve. *Grief Unseen* by Laura Seftel is a lovely book which goes into pregnancy loss using the power of the arts to heal. Dr Christiane Northrup's book *Women's Bodies, Women's Wisdom* (2009) gives good insight into all aspects of pregnancy and includes a section on Pregnancy Loss (page 479). I have incorporated exercises in the creative section of this book that will support the expression and release of difficult feelings.

   + **All of my feelings are Safe (B. A. Dansby)**

Healing Pregnancy Loss – Abortion

I think it is only fair to mention the subject of Abortion as it is widely on the increase and often leaves emotional scars that can last a lifetime. It is a 'loss' even though the pregnancy may not have been wanted. I want to stress that I am not here to judge or take sides as a woman's reproductive choice is her business.

In *Women's Bodies, Women's Wisdom*, Dr Northrup discusses abortion and female fertility with a depth of understanding gained by her extensive experience in her medical career. She suggests abortion can be 'unfinished business' for many women and stresses that it is a very complex issue. Women taking control over their reproduction is very empowering and threatens the whole patriarchal system so it comes as no surprise that it has always been a hot topic for political debate. Historically, abortion has been shrouded with guilt and shame because it is assumed that conception is the negligent responsibility of the woman not the co-operative co-creation of a man and a woman. Northrup discusses the breakthrough for women's sexual freedom and how many women simulate male sexual behaviour that does not always entail conception consequences.

There were nearly 190,000 abortions in England and Wales in 2010 (Department of Health Statistics) and 42 million worldwide (Centre for Bio-Ethical Reform). This is a high number.

One thing is certain; abortion should not be used as a form of contraception because it has long lasting emotional reverberations not to mention the unpleasant ordeal that a woman goes through. Sexual freedom comes with responsibility.

About half of women who have an abortion will have considered their choices, talked it over with professionals and come to their conclusions consciously. It is never a straightforward decision and there are many reasons for choosing this option. In most cases, a woman's feelings will be suppressed, whether they are aware of this or not, in order to make the decision that they feel is right. The other half of women will be in total denial that this procedure will have any effect on them at all. The sad fact is that often, amongst younger women or teenagers, an abortion is performed because of carelessness in taking contraceptive precautions before having sex.

When a woman is then ready to have a child, it can be really valuable to allow all the 'true' feelings to surface. This does not mean the original decision is undermined but new feelings can emerge. Abortion is a loss which deserves to be grieved like any other loss and the woman given all the love and support she needs.

Expressing honestly how we feel about our abortion through art, writing, poetry or sculpture can once again remove any historical emotional barriers to free the way, especially for a wanted birth. For example, there may be unresolved anger at a previous partner. Northrup says, 'with decades of guilt and shame as an emotional backdrop, however, many women never adequately process the emotional aspects of abortion' (Northrup, C. 2009). There are exercises for releasing emotional trauma related to abortion in the Creative section of this book. My desire is for women to be able to talk about and process their sexual experiences, without guilt or shame, to live life authentically, and be loved and supported by their global Sisters.

Sexual Abuse and Rape

Survivors of sexual abuse or rape can experience hospital birth with its inevitable interventions, or interventions per se, as another violation of their body. Natural childbirth can be a way of reclaiming your once damaged body into an empowering experience, but you will need extra support. There are 25-40% of women in the UK who have been sexually abused (although it is hard to determine) but who do not necessarily present high risk symptoms (Furin, K., 2005) and therefore do not receive the positive attention they need.

Sheila Kitzinger (*Birth Crisis*, 2007) and Dr Christiane Northrup (*Women's Bodies, Women's Wisdom*, 2009) write about sexual abuse and its potential effect on pregnancy and birth in a very sensitive and well informed way.

By following the empowering tools in this book you will be able to work through some of the issues that might still be buried in the unconscious. Affirming your 'Innocence' is profoundly beneficial under these circumstances. Having extra support from a therapist can also be very helpful.

⬥ I am the innocent child of a Gentle God (B. A. Dansby)

It is definitely possible to have a pleasurable birth after experiencing any form of abuse. You can do this by entering into the process of conception, pregnancy and birth with an open mind and a commitment to inner work which will undoubtedly impact positively on your experience.

*   *   *

Pregnancy loss from whichever perspective requires healing, love, understanding and much patience, most of all towards the mother but also the family and an understanding from society in general. This is why the so called 'hormonal emotions' during pregnancy, as described usually by men but also by some women, are often nothing to do with hormone imbalances but due to unexpressed issues or unresolved experiences which manifest in erratic behaviour or unfounded emotions. I am not saying it is nothing to do with hormones but not if we use them as our scapegoat to brush over our real feelings. Similar to menstruation, our ability to mask what we really feel becomes virtually impossible, so whatever comes up during menstruation or pregnancy/birth is a sign of the deeper reality within and can act as a useful compass towards greater self realisation and healing. Art can be a valuable tool for this healing process.

Unleash Your Creativity

Art Exercises for Self Empowerment

Self Empowering Tools for Conception to Birth and Beyond

The exercises in this chapter will allow you to gain deeper insight into your thoughts and feelings about your desire for conception, pregnancy, birth and about becoming a parent. You will discover positive ways to overcome any unnecessary obstacles towards greater clarity and a more pleasurable experience. The following list suggests helpful practices to support yourself through conception, pregnancy, birth and beyond.

- Affirmations - turn life-diminishing thoughts into positive daily thoughts

- Breathe deeply and fully, exercise gently and eat healthily

- Communicate – express any thoughts and feelings to clear the way

- Draw, paint, sculpt, photograph, craft. Write: poetry, stories or just write a stream of consciousness

- Educate – read lots of positive stories/books and surround yourself with positive people

- Flow – relax and make space to engage with your pregnancy and rest as much as possible

- Give way to visualisation. What mood would you like to create around your birth?

'Your vision will become clear only when you can look into your own heart. Who looks outside, dreams; who looks inside, awakes' (Jung, C., cited in Elias, J., & Ketcham, K. (1996) *In the House of the Moon – Reclaiming the Feminine Spirit of Healing*).

It is really important NOT to judge yourself if you express things that may appear negative to you as you unlock unnecessary thoughts and feelings that may stand in the way of your liberation! Once these are freed, they no longer need to be repressed so do not be alarmed. If, however, you are feeling particularly overwhelmed or in need of support from a counsellor or art therapist then it may be helpful to find someone locally, speak to a trustworthy friend, or you can have an online session with me either by email or Skype™. Check out the website for more information www.theartofbirth.co.uk.

I once drew a picture of my mother on the delivery table with blood spewing out of her vagina and gushing out of the room. When I was born I was put in a cradle far away from my mother and cried all night which, she told me years later, gave her a headache. This made me feel guilty all my life, and at a deep level made me wish I had never been born to save my mother that agony. I had to clear this mental picture from my psyche to cleanse an aspect of my birth story. It is not that I judged my mother and made her 'wrong', I had been fed a story that needed to be expressed in order for me to heal. Once I expressed the story, it freed the way to a more positive relationship with my mother. It is also interesting that I never once thought what it must have been like for me, a newly born baby, to be separated from my mother for many hours after birth without any attention or skin-to-skin contact.

A client of mine painted a picture of mountains, flowers and a bright sun. She was unsure about how it related to her pregnancy but realised the scene made her feel good and happy. It was a kind of spiritual talisman as she was very connected to nature and this was a place, albeit a fictional place, where she felt most at peace and 'on top of the world'. She was having some trouble with her partner and this picture acted as a positive container for her – a self soothing mechanism. Further pictures were much more spontaneous and playful.

The aim is to have fun and build a relationship with your body and mind because it will open up a whole new world of possibilities that will enable you to experience your pregnancy and birth in a profound way. The exercises in this book can support every woman (and man) in many different ways. Essentially, birth will be what it will be and that is OK.

Materials

Most of the materials below can be bought very cheaply in shops like Hobby Craft, or even the 99p shop (in the UK). You can start with some paper and pencils if money is short and build up gradually. Art shops or online stores offer better quality art materials for the more experienced or adventurous creator. Suggested materials to use:

⬇ Paper and Card

> White paper in sketch-pad form or loose sheets. A4 is standard size or A3 can also be cut into smaller pieces. Pack or individual sheets of coloured paper are fun too. Any size is fine!

Pencils and Rubber

Lead pencils or coloured pencils. You can often buy them in boxes of different colours

Pastels

Soft chalk pastels and/or oil pastels, charcoal, fixer (a cheap hairspray can be used instead)

Crayons

Boxes of mixed colours

Felt Tip Pens

These can be bought in most stationers or even supermarkets and can be fun to doodle with

Paint Brushes

Various sizes and you can buy these in packs with the different size brushes

Paints

Water colour, Gouache, Acrylic (or Oil if you feel inspired *check the labels of the oil paints first as some colours can be toxic). The basic colours you will need are: white, black, blue, red, yellow, green, purple, brown, orange and others if you like. You can buy boxes with all sorts of colours or you can choose individual colours, in addition to the basic ones, as you desire. www.Stockmar.de water colour paints are lovely for wet on wet or veil painting

Palette

You can buy plastic palettes, books of disposable palette sheets, or you can be creative and use plastic plates, aluminium takeaway containers, or plastic lids such as Margarine tubs

Glue

PVA or Prit Stick is good to start with

- Scissors

- Masking Tape

- Accessories

  Ruler, glitter, sequins, large jar or plastic container like a yoghurt pot for water for your brushes, sponge for wiping, tissue for dabbing brushes.

- Clay

  You can buy packets of brown or grey clay in craft shops

- Magazines for collage

- Recycled Items

  Anything from pieces of fabric, to wool, tissue paper, or any object for making fun 'things'.

A Note Before you Start:

It is a good idea to set out a selection of your art materials (paint, paint brushes, pastels, pencils, pencil sharpener and rubber, clay, mixed media items) and paper with a jar of water and cloth BEFORE you start your art exercise. It is useful to have as many materials as you can so you are free to be spontaneous and choose what you desire in the moment when you feel ready to start. You may also wish to do a relaxation process before you begin (see below).

Don't worry if your materials are limited, you can create with the most basic materials.

You may also wish to buy a special book or journal for writing or doodling.

Please note: when I say make an 'image', this can mean 2D or 3D and in any media. It also means you can make more than one image.

When I say 'find a space that is free from noise or distraction', I understand that this is not always very easy... just be inventive.

When I invite you to 'tune in' and 'see what comes up' this may not happen straight away so don't worry. It can take time to get used to the art-making process.

You do not need to do ALL of the exercises, pick and choose as you wish.

At any point you may wish to ask yourself two simple questions:

- What do I want to Express right now?

- What is my Baby trying to Communicate to me? (You are co-creating a Life)

General Self Development Exercises

For:

Women

Pregnant women

Fathers/Partners

Parents

Midwives, Doulas, Doctors

Child Birth Educators

Teenagers, Elders

Everyone

Why meditation or relaxation exercises? Meditation/relaxation exercises help you to quieten your mind and go within, disconnecting you from your busy mind. They reduce stress and enable you to ground yourself from the busyness of daily life and find a still place where you can gently allow your deeper thoughts and feelings to surface. It is not compulsory to do these exercises before you start, but taking a moment to centre yourself can be helpful. You can also use your own relaxation technique, CD, meditation or centring process.

Relaxation Exercise - Centring Process

This relaxation technique can be used before you embark on any one of the following creative exercises as a centring process, or purely for relaxation. If it is possible, find a quiet space. You may wish to light a candle, or play very gentle and relaxing music of your choice.

- Sitting or lying down, however you feel most comfortable, close your eyes if this feels right. With your mouth slightly open, relax your jaw and open your throat. Take some full breaths – deep yet gentle; inhale and exhale.

- While you are breathing rhythmically in and out, start by relaxing the muscles in your eyes, nose, mouth, jaw, head and the back of your neck.

- Relax the tension in your shoulders and down your arms. Then slowly move your focus down your spine, relax your buttocks and your genitals. Feel the support beneath you whether you are sitting or lying down.

- Relax your chest, your solar plexus, and your belly (and be aware of your baby's presence).

- Release the tension in your thighs, your knees, your calves, your ankles, all the way down to your feet and let any tension out through your toes.

- Take some more deep breaths and allow all the tension to just melt away as this is your time to be with YOU and everything is taken care of right here, right now.

- Know that YOU are welcome in this moment and anything you wish to express is welcome too, however new you are to unlocking your creativity. And remember, your being is innocent and it is safe and acceptable to feel ALL of your feelings.

- Take some time to just let go and breathe, allow thoughts to drift in and out, not paying too much attention to them and relax.

- Then bringing your awareness back to the room and with your eyes still closed, wriggle your fingers and toes, yawn and stretch your arms and legs.

- When you feel ready, you may ask yourself the very gentle, non specific question:

- 'What do I need to express?'

- Take a deep breath and lightly hold the palms of your hands over your eyes. When you are ready, slowly open your eyes. In your own time, move your hands and adjust yourself to the light. When you feel ready, begin your chosen exercise.

Take a Breath – for Release and Relaxation

(Inspired by SOURCE Process & Breathwork by Binnie A. Dansby)

This is another great way to relax both your mind and body and increase wellbeing.

- Find a comfortable place to sit or lie down and remember to keep warm.

- Close your eyes if that feels comfortable, relax your jaw and open your throat. Having an open throat will relax the cervix, as they are linked, so it is also important to remember this during labour.

- Take a deep breath and have a big yawn.

- Breathe rhythmically in and out, gently connecting your breath as you breathe: this means that there are no pauses between the in and out breath – it is circular.

- If you have funny sensations in your body, don't worry as this is the breath releasing any unwanted energy. Sometimes people get pins and needles, stiff fingers and hands, involuntary movements, tears, etc so just affirm that your body is safe.

- Let any thoughts drift in and out, there is no need to give them any attention right now. This is your time to just be with your breath and to relax with your baby.

- During your breathing session, gently hold the word 'Yes' in your mind. And 'Yes, I can do it' and even say this out aloud. The word 'Yes' also opens your throat and gives you a positive affirmation.

- Breathe for as long as you feel comfortable, gently and rhythmically, without strain or goal achieving. Think 'Yes' and repeat 'Yes' and/or 'Yes I can do it'.

- When you feel ready – and this can be 5, 10, 15, 20 minutes – begin to breathe normally and wiggle your toes, have a good stretch and bring your awareness back to the room.

- You may wish to use some art materials and make an image of anything that came up for you. You may also wish to write in your journal.

- Otherwise you can move on to an exercise of your choice.

Daily Doodle

(Warm Up Exercise – For everyone)

This is a great exercise to begin with as it allows one to draw freely without any purpose except making a lot of scribbles or marks on the paper. It aims to give your mind a rest and enter into the realm of spontaneity. It can also help to release any inhibitions if you are not sure how to begin an exercise. This exercise can come before any other exercise.

Begin by sitting, either at a table or on the floor (wherever you feel most comfortable and inspired). Feel your body sink into the chair or the floor. Take a few deep breaths and you may wish to make a noise on the out breath to really let out any tension. Remind yourself gently that this is your special time to be creative and that all that you express is welcome.

- Preferably sit with your eyes closed (but open is ok if this feels more comfortable) and for about 30 seconds let a pen, pencil or crayon wander aimlessly over the page, or 'take a line for a walk' (as the well known artists Paul Klee once said). Just make spontaneous marks, lines, scribbles, doodles. Try not to 'think' about what you are doing, be spontaneous.

- Open your eyes and see if you can find an image or pattern amongst the scribbles. Sometimes a figure, an animal or a particular shape jumps out at you, but don't worry if it doesn't. Just have a go and see what happens. You can try it several times.

    Then, if you wish, develop it further by perhaps colouring it in. Do whatever you feel and you may be astonished at the result.

It is a chance for you to express your inner thoughts, feelings and emotions without censoring the outcome.

Finally, sit back and ponder on your image.

Does anything come to mind?

Does the image have a particular 'feeling' or 'theme'?

Explore any possibilities. It may have just been a fun warm-up exercise.

The Secret Book – Writing for fun

(For everyone)

This is a great way to uncover your hidden thoughts and feelings by spontaneous, free writing – some people call it stream of consciousness because there are no pauses for your intellectual mind to step in and edit. It is always wonderful when you give your imagination permission to say whatever comes into your head first.

Buy a special book which you can decorate yourself if you fancy which can be used as your 'secret writing book'. This is private for you and your thoughts.

    Begin by sitting, either at a table or on the floor, sofa, bed (wherever you feel most comfortable and inspired). Feel your body sink into the chair or wherever you are sitting. Take a few deep breaths and you may wish to make a noise on the out breath to really let out any tension. Remind yourself gently that this is your special time to be creative and all of your expression is welcome.

    Take a pen or pencil and start writing anything that comes into your head. Do not judge what comes out and keep going, without stopping, until you've written at least 2 pages or for about 5 minutes.

When you have finished, you may read through your writing and see if there are any themes that emerge. You may spot a recurring word, sentence or theme. Ponder over it and see if it speaks to you in any way. You may write these thoughts in your journal too and illustrate them or even make an image if this feels appropriate.

Dream Diary

(For everyone)

This is a great exercise to do every morning.

You may treat yourself to a special 'Dream Diary' book which you can decorate however you fancy or you can use your journal. Keep it by your bed with a pen or pencil and as soon as you wake up in the morning and still in that half asleep/half awake state, notice any dreams you had in the night. Again you will be able to build up a picture of what your dreams are expressing.

Look at any recurring themes, images or symbols. What do they mean to you? There is no need to consult a dream interpretation book as you will begin to discover what your dreams mean to you personally.

If some of your dreams seem negative or characters are sinister or threatening perhaps, remember that dreams are often 'metaphors' for feelings or situations and similarly people in dreams may often represent aspects of our own self.

Me, Myself and I

(For everyone)

A self portrait can be a good place to start because it enables us to get to know how we feel about ourselves. Many clues lie within our interpretation of self identity. Getting to know the inner 'you' will support you to transform any aspect that is not a celebration of the fabulous person that you are and heal any life diminishing perceptions.

Set out a selection of your art materials. I would suggest you use a pastel, crayon or pencil to start with but other materials of your choice are also fine

Sit quietly at the table or on the floor and centre yourself.

- If you wish, you can do the centring process or otherwise scan your body and relax any parts that need it and take some deep breaths feeling the support beneath you.

- There are different ways to approach the self portrait so here is a list for you to choose from (you don't have to do them all):

- Sit in front of a mirror and with a pencil, crayon or pastel do a quick 2 minute portrait without worrying about your technical skill.

- Touch your face and draw what you feel without looking in the mirror.

- Close your eyes and draw your face.

- Draw your face with your opposite hand (i.e. if you are right handed then use your left).

- Draw a picture of your face or body purely from your memory (no mirrors).

- Make a clay model of your face and or body. Try touching your face with your eyes closed first and see what comes up and then you can try it with eyes open but from memory.

- Finally you can draw, paint, model, collage, or use mixed media to make a portrait of your face using a mirror. It can also be any size.

- You may also wish to try this exercise using your whole nude body (not just the face).

What came up for you?

How do you see yourself or feel about yourself? This could be in general or how you perceive yourself today in this moment.

How do you see yourself as the 'parent' or the 'professional' you, or the 'partner'? You may wish to write down your thoughts and feelings in your journal.

How is your inner perception of yourself? How do you 'see' yourself today? How are you feeling?

What is rising up and wanting to be expressed?

What is my baby trying to communicate to me through this exercise?

This can reveal your current self-perception and can be a reflective experience. Try not to judge how you perceive yourself because you are fabulous just the way you are now.

Other exercises:

✦ Claim Your Name

Take your name; this can be your first name, abbreviated name, nickname, surname or even a fantasy name and write it down on the paper which you can decorate, illustrate, manipulate or embellish in any way you like.

✦ What Am I

Draw yourself as either an object or something from nature like a tree, river, rock, plant, flower, animal, building, a landscape, or represent yourself as a particular colour or shape. It is also possible to include them in some kind of landscape, cityscape or seascape.

✦ Picture Me

Find some old magazines and cut or rip out any pictures that are appropriate or significant to you right now. Make a collage about your life: you could try one of your past, one of your present feelings about parenthood and one of your desired or 'ideal' future.

Other options could be cutting out words to describe how you are feeling or even find one statement which sums up your life now.

✦ The Family Portrait

You can use any media for this project and it can be about your family growing up and/or your current family (even if you just have a partner and no children yet).

You can start with simply portraying your family either in a realistic way or a symbolic or abstract way. You can then portray your family as an object or as an animal, or something in nature like plants or trees or anything else you can think of and have some fun!

You can also make a collage of your family by cutting out images from magazines that represent or remind you of your family members in some way – whether alive or deceased. Why not try to depict your family line? (I.e. the female family line: you, mother, grandmother, great grandmother, or historical female family members you have heard about in conversation. Men can represent their masculine line).

⬥ Reflect on your images:

Afterwards, look at your image and just observe it with an open mind for a moment. Do any symbolic clues jump out? Is the image big or small, light or dark, to the left or to the right, what are the proportions like, how do you fit into your particular landscape? Again please don't judge, just note what is being presented to you for your own enlightenment. What intuitive message is it whispering to you? Take some time to digest whatever has filtered to the surface and remember that any release of emotion is a good thing and be gentle with yourself.

Your Inner Child

(For everyone)

Your inner child relates to your different stages of childhood up to puberty. At any point during this time you could have had difficult experiences which stay buried in your subconscious until they are healed. Looking back at memories and exploring their meaning can be very enlightening and help to ease the burden you may be carrying without realising it.

It is quite useful to explore your childhood memories of fear, loss, disappointment, joy, good things, bad things, funny events, relationship i.e. with siblings or with parents, embarrassment, shame, happy or unhappy moments to see what they reveal. Any repressed memories from childhood can become activated during pregnancy and birth or even when trying to conceive, or when one is already a parent. Unearthing and expelling any repressed thought, feeling or memory will leave you free to move forward with your life.

In these exercises you can use any art, craft, mixed media material, clay or anything you fancy. It is time to become a child!

- You may wish to do one of the centring processes to get you into your body. Alternatively you can listen to your favourite music to get you into your creative zone.

- Start by tuning into your first or earliest memory and make an image. Try not to judge what comes up and let your imagination run free.

Additional Themes – Make an Image about any of the following:

- Choose a memory that is either positive or negative.

- Tune into an embarrassing moment in your childhood that made you feel ashamed.

- Think back to things you were not allowed to have in childhood, or something you were not allowed to be or do.

- Can you remember the first memory of significant separation?

- Recall a particular event.

- Think of a time you experienced a Loss.

- Did you have any Secrets, whether this was a guilty secret or a fun secret? Family secrets, for example, can be very stressful for a child.

- How was religion handled in your family when you were a child? Can you think of a specific memory related in some way to religion?

- Can you think of recurring thought patterns you inherited that were quite dominant?

- Draw objects related to childhood memories.

- Make an image of a person you disliked.

- Make an image of a teacher – one you liked and one you disliked.

- Recall a best friend and make an image of him/her.

- Tell a story about your childhood in a cartoon strip.

- Make an image of a popular super hero/heroine that you identified with as a child.

- Paint with your hands (finger painting) or even with your feet (make sure you have some form of cleaning equipment close at hand)! Making a mess can be very liberating but also very activating, so gently take note of your feelings as you do it.

Reflect on your images:

Once again, observe your images without judgement but also take note of any judgements that may surface. Notice what emerges when you choose a topic. Which ones did you instinctually gravitate towards? What came up spontaneously? If you uncovered some very painful memories do allow yourself to grieve. Tears for the loss of a situation is really helpful even if you think it is unworthy of grieving. Let it out and let it go. If you unearth memories that are too difficult for you to process on your own or in a group, do consult a therapist, or find suitable support. Otherwise you are welcome to email me at: alex@theartofbirth.co.uk

Lotus Meditation

(For women)

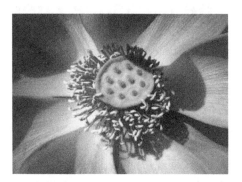

Close up of Lotus Flower – photograph by Alexandra Florschutz

Find a comfortable place. Sit or lie down, whatever makes you feel relaxed and safe. Play some relaxing, soothing music which creates a sense of well being for you.

- Allow yourself to drift off and call into your imagination a Lotus Flower.

- Picture its centre, the heart of the flower, circular with little raised spots at regular intervals. Mull over this being like the womb, origin, source and vulva.

- Surrounding this 'womb' centre are lots of protective sepals or stamen. These are like many layers of protection, whether physical or spiritual. Gently experience them as support emanating from all the people in your life.

- Then let the imagination wander to the outstretched petals, in all their beauty and splendour, for lady lotus is not making any apologies for being open and free to the world, for she is innocent and at the same time sexually radiant in full bloom. Let this sit with you until it envelopes every part of your being.

⟁ Once you feel ready, wriggle your toes and fingers and bring your attention back to the room. Have a good stretch and yawn and give yourself a hug to feel your body and ground yourself once more. When you are ready open your eyes.

⟁ You may wish to savour the experience and write any thoughts or experiences in your journal.

⟁ You may feel inspired to select some appropriate art materials that you feel drawn to and make an image on whatever came up for you. How do you perceive yourself after this meditation?

The Pleasure Diet

(For women – men can also do their own version)

This is the ONLY diet you ever really need to go on in your life!

⟁ List five things you are going to do for yourself this week that will either nurture you, inspire you or just be lots of fun! This list can be endless and unique to the individual. Take a luxurious bubble bath at an unusual time, make yourself a meal fit for a goddess, buy yourself flowers, a present, watch a movie you have always wanted to see, have a coffee and read a magazine or favourite book, do something arty, give yourself a manicure and/or pedicure (or get someone else to do it), have a massage, etc.

⟁ Write a letter to your divine Feminine and tell her how wonderful you are and how much you love her. Tell her that you are listening to her. See what comes back to you.

⟁ Write or doodle in your journal while thinking pleasurable thoughts or listening to some pleasurable music.

Creative Dancing

(For everyone)

Choose music that really inspires you and makes your heart sing or you connect to the vibe. In your own time simply move in any way you desire. Dance like nobody's watching as they say. Dance as though you are ten years old. You may wish to do some warm up stretches beforehand if this feels right. Try and tune into your body and move in a way that feels comfortable to you (especially when you are pregnant) and feel the energy shift. This is a great exercise to do when you feel a bit tired, edgy, stuck, afraid or just want to have some fun!

Self Celebrations

(Mainly for women – but men are also welcome to do this exercise)

List ten things daily you think you have done really well. This could be taking some time out to relax during a busy day, standing up to the boss, expressing yourself clearly, noticing the beauty of your favourite flower, winning first prize, getting an upgrade and so on. Anything, however big or small, that you feel is some kind of self achievement. The more you do this the more the list will grow and you will begin to experience yourself as a creator.

I know this can be challenging for a lot of women because we are raised in a society which says it is not good to brag or be full of ourselves. Then we get to secondary school and beyond and have to learn how to do 'self assessments' where we have to 'sing our praises'! Why don't we just sing our praises from the beginning and love every big or small achievement we do or have done. Why not start now and see your abundance grow.

Appreciations

(Mainly for women – but men are also welcome to do this exercise)

List ten things daily you are grateful for and, again, they can be big or small. The more you focus on the good in your life the more you will realise how much you have already. This gives the feeling of our inner cup being full as opposed to empty. And once again, focussing on the positives in your life will make them multiply. Recognition is often the first step. This will be supportive at any point on the journey from conception to birth and beyond.

Wish Lists

(Mainly for women – but men are also welcome to do this exercise)

This is a list of everything you wish, desire or fancy whether it is to have a day off, have great sex with your partner, or learn to play an instrument, buy that new dress, feel adored, have an amazing birth or a good night's sleep! Make a list of at least ten wishes and add to it daily. Post it on the fridge if you feel like it so people can fulfil your desires if they can. It will make them feel good to help you too. It will also tune you into yourself even more.

Wish Boards

(For everyone)

Find magazines, newspapers, anything that has pictures and words that you can use to cut out and express all your wishes visually.

- Start by finding a good size piece of cardboard, a canvas or board canvas. You will need your PVA glue, an old paintbrush, a container for the glue, such as a used plastic pot, and scissors.

- After doing a relaxation process, ask yourself the gentle question: 'What do I need to express right now?'

- Just flick through the magazines and cut out any picture or word that seems to 'speak' to you.

- Once you have collected a good amount, lay them on the board or canvas in a very spontaneous way. You don't need to think too deeply or analyse what you are putting where at this stage. Review your layout and see if any image needs to be moved and then you can use the glue to stick them into place.

- When you have finished, stand back and look at your wish board.

- Ask yourself:

Is there a theme running through the pictures?

Are there any recurring images or words that mean something to you?

What is your heart trying to reveal to you about your deep desires or wishes?

You may wish to make notes in your journal.

Nature Reflections

(For parents, children, anyone)

Follow the seasons and collect the gifts that Mother Nature offers for a Nature Table.

Walk in Nature as often as possible and breathe in the fresh air. If you live in a city, try and find a park or take some trips to the countryside, or observe the changing seasons of the ocean.

It can be wonderful to follow the seasons with a 'Nature Table' which can be changed throughout the year and keeps you connected to the cycles of the year. A nature table is simply a space on which you place a cloth of some kind and decorate it with things you find in nature or other seasonal appropriate objects (e.g. at Easter, if you celebrate this festival, I put a tray on top of a particular work surface in my kitchen and cover it with moss I collect from my garden. I use a little flat pottery dish concealed in the moss and fill it with water to resemble a pond. I put a branch with leaf buds in a vase and hang various size decorated eggs on it. I then place different objects, either found in nature, or little things I've bought or collected over the years like small yellow chicks, crystals, rabbits, mini candles. Things that suggest new life, joy and love).

An art exercise:

- Sitting quietly, tune into the current Season. What is the weather like? Is it warm or cold? Is there much daylight?

- Choose your materials that feel appropriate and make an image of this season. See what it reveals to you.

- You can also sit and contemplate on the seasons and pick one that you feel needs expressing. Imagine a scene in nature and make an image in any material.

- Once you have finished, you may wish to ask yourself some questions:

Which season did you choose and why?

Is there anything about the scene or the colours which have a significance and why?

What is the mood of the picture?

Are there any people in it and if so what are they doing? Who do they represent?

What do the colours you chose represent?

If you have drawn/painted a tree, does it have leaves, is it bare, does it have roots that go into the earth or is it floating in the air?

You may wish to jot down notes in your journal on anything that comes to mind.

There is no right or wrong way, just information.

Your Story – Autobiography

(For everyone)

Write, draw, paint or sculpt your life story so far.

It may be easier to start by writing it down and then progress to image making.

🔸 Begin with *your birth story* as it was told to you – or how you experienced it if you have that kind of insight.

Put pen to paper and let it run away with you and don't stop and think or edit, just stream of consciousness or free flow writing. If emotions come to the surface – they usually do – just let them happen and express them knowing that 'all of my feelings are safe and acceptable'. What you feel in any given moment is the right way to feel so just let it be. Relax and take a breath. Tears are only grief, a letting go of energy that has often been stored up for years.

🔸 Then write your childhood story as it was told to you.

🔸 Finally, write about your childhood as you remember it. Please don't judge yourself about how you perceive your experience. I give you permission to say it how you think it was, in your opinion. Whether you think you 'should not' say something or question if it was 'really true' or not, it is ok. It is the way YOU experienced it and that is what matters now.

When you have finished and allowed yourself to digest its contents. See if you can find any themes that have emerged. Themes such as – I was always trying to help others because that was the only time my parents seemed to praise me and the only time I was considered a 'good girl'. So thought patterns evolved such as 'I'm not good enough', 'my energy is too much for people', 'I am doing it wrong', 'I have to please others to be liked'. I have discovered, in later years, that these thought patterns are fairly archetypal.

Once you have identified themes or patterns, can you discover any 'thought patterns' that you have been carrying since childhood? There will probably be many, so list them all. Start with ten but if you go over, that is fine. Everyone will have lots, even the most enlightened and the most sorted of us! It is not something to be ashamed of; just a way of identifying the mind's conditioning which can be changed at any time.

Out of these thought patterns there will arise a handful of 'archetypal' or 'foundation' thought patterns. Write these down. It is what all your thoughts boil down to – the base line. Mine was 'I am doing it wrong'! Everything seemed to stem from that powerful thought! When you have one or two thought patterns see how you can change them to a positive affirmation. 'I am doing it wrong' became 'I am innocent' (an innocent child of a gentle god/goddess which is one of Dansby's Archetypal Affirmations). So any time I am triggered into a feeling of 'not good enough' (luckily doesn't happen too often nowadays) I just say 'thank you' and 'I am innocent'. That immediately puts me back in touch with the positive reality – not the negative one. Let me explain Innocence a little deeper. For example, if I get angry and smash a plate, I am kind of responsible for that but if it is an old childhood feeling where I had been unnecessarily criticised, then I can assume my innocence as a baby is born innocent and full of love. It doesn't mean that I don't take responsibility for my actions. The essence of who I am is Innocent. (More examples on p168).

- ♣ You can choose some art materials that you are drawn to and make images of scenes that come into your head, or you may wish to interpret some of your thought patterns visually.

- ♣ When you have finished, you can review and see what speaks to you in this visual language.

Life Lines

(For everyone)

Drawing, painting or illustrating our Life Line can also be enlightening and this is another way of charting our biography.

- ♣ Choose fairly large paper – probably white but you can use other colours.

- ♣ Start with a line across the paper – your time line. It can be a straight line or it can be a line like an aerial view of a meandering river, or mountainous peaks with your life's ups and downs. Allow the peaks and valleys of your life be revealed before your eyes.

- ♣ Divide the line into equal 7 yearly intervals: 0-7, 7-14, 14-21, 21-28, etc. Follow by making marks on the line where specific or important or memorable things happened in your life. Once again do not judge what comes into consciousness, just allow them to emerge.

- ♣ You can write the memory, make a short poem, draw a doodle, collage or however you are inspired to portray these events.

- ♣ Step back and take a look at the 'highlights' of your life. Are you surprised? How do you feel? What is the overall mood?

- ♣ If you like, you can then make an image that expresses this mood. Be gentle with yourself and know that your feelings are better expressed than repressed.

Keep a journal of doodles and snippets of thoughts, poems or affirmations that arise out of any of these exercises.

Mandalas

(For everyone)

Mandala is a Sanskrit word meaning a sacred Circle. Circles are archetypal forms found in all aspects of life such as water, plants, the universe, the womb; circles represent a safe container or the concept of eternity. In Psychology, the circle is thought to be the gateway to the unconscious part of our Self. Carl Jung used Mandalas to access deeper emotions that lay buried in his unconscious realm and, by making visual representations of these repressed feelings; he was able to affect positive change. The circle is seen as a container which holds the emotional contents safely within its boundaries. Jung referred to the circle as the symbol of the feminine and to the square as the symbol of the masculine, both of which live within each human being (Anima/Animus). The colours, forms and structures of Tibetan Mandalas related to inner states of consciousness and the circle within a square is indicative of total balance.

- There are different ways to approach a Mandala so feel free to experiment. Start with white paper (it is easier to start with white until you get more comfortable with the process). I would suggest A3 size paper to begin with and then you can play with different sizes and colours, especially black.

- Before you begin, it is helpful to do the centring process as this will take you within yourself and begin to loosen your imagination ready for making your Mandala.

- The first Mandala: Draw a circle on your paper with a compass or by drawing around a dinner plate.

- Select your desired materials. You may choose to draw or paint inside the circle.

- Put an arrow on the back of the picture to indicate which way up it is.

- The second Mandala: Draw a small circle in the middle of the paper about the size of a pea. You can use a lead pencil, a coloured pencil or a pen.

- Sit quietly and clear your mind from the busyness of the day. Think of a shape like an S, a line about half a centimetre, a triangle and so on and jot it down on the right hand side of the paper at the bottom for your reference. Then draw this shape around the centre circle. You will now have a small central circle with S shapes radiating out from the outer edge of the circle.

- Think of another shape; jot it down on the right hand side above the first S shape. Now draw that shape on top of the S shape all the way round.

- You can build up your Mandala in this way and remember to spontaneously think of a shape, jot it down on the right hand side and then proceed to add it to the shape before on the Mandala. Try not to think about it too much but let your imagination speak to you freely – follow your Self.

- Once you have created the desired size of your Mandala, you can colour it in whatever way you like.

- Keep a Mandala Journal. This can be an amazing way to capture your thoughts.

- Feelings, insights and energy within a safe circular space.

- You can also give your Mandalas a title as this offers another dimension for self realisation.

- Once you have completed your Mandala, sit back and look at it (or them) for a while.

Ask yourself the question: What is my Mandala trying to reveal to me? Make notes in your journal too if you feel like doing so. It is interesting to look back at the journey.

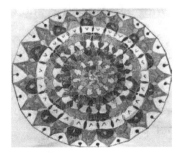

A Mandala Doodle by Alex Florschutz
(This was built up from the centre with no compass or plate to create the circle effect).

Making a Mess

(For everyone)

Having a baby is a rather messy experience so it can be very helpful to learn how to make a mess and get your hands dirty before you have a baby. We live very busy and controlled lives where order overrules chaos. It is very liberating to relinquish our self control and revel in the tactile freedom of the art materials.

- Time to get down and dirty! Get out the poster paints, the clay or any tactile media and role up your sleeves. If you have a roll of paper (such as a roll of plain wallpaper), spread out a large amount of it on the floor (if possible, or even outside) and tape down the edges or secure them with heavy objects.

- It is time to give yourself permission to 'go for it'! No more self restraint, forget being clean and tidy, let go of being in control and most importantly... Have FUN!

- You may wish to put on some music that gets you going, revs you up or inspires you in some way.

- Dive into the experience... You can squirt the paint straight onto the paper, or use large brushes and paint fast and furiously. Feel free to mix the paint on the paper. You can even use your fingers and hands or feet to paint with! Have a bowl of water and an old towel nearby for when you finish!

What feelings does it bring up?

Did you feel out of control or liberated?

Does your picture have a name?

What colours are dominant?

What do these colours symbolise?

Are there any motifs that you wish to develop in another picture?

Jot down your thoughts and feelings in your journal.

The Rainbow

(For everyone)

Working with colour helps to relieve anxiety and can be very soothing and healing. It penetrates our essence or soul. We experience the most stunning colours in the rainbow. One could say that the whole colour spectrum in its purest form is reflected in the sky which penetrates our whole spiritual being.

'Our whole physiology experiences this colour world, not only our eyes. The rainbow is particularly significant in that it creates a bridge, both metaphorically and physically. It is a bridge spanning heaven and earth, its beauty providing a harmonious sense experience. It can also lead us into a meditative mood giving harmony and balance for the soul' (Lord, A., 2010 *Colour Dynamics – workbook for watercolour painting and colour theory*).

The Colours of the Rainbow are Red, Orange, Yellow, Green, Blue, Indigo and Violet which are the colours you see in the sky in the rainbow, or when you look through a prism or a clear crystal. The rainbow is a reflection of all the colours of the universe. They become visible through light, air and water – sun and rain.

- Try to use good quality paper if you can. This can be heavy drawing paper, cartridge paper, watercolour paper, a spiral watercolour book, or even a roll of medium-weight wallpaper/lining paper (not pre pasted of course!).

- You will need a place to make the paper wet like the sink or bath/shower.

- Use a sponge to remove excess water and an appropriate work surface such as a painting board, a table or the floor. Have a jar of water handy for cleaning your brush.

- Watercolour paints. You can buy tubes of these and I recommend you buy the basics: Red, Yellow, Ultramarine Blue, Prussian Blue and Violet/Purple but you can always buy Orange and Green if you prefer not to mix the colours. In case you are not sure: mixing red and yellow makes orange, mixing blue and yellow makes green and mixing red and (ultramarine) blue makes purple. Dilute each colour with a little water in your palette or recycled pots.

- Before you begin, just take a moment and note how you are feeling.

- Apply a wash of colour in an arc across the paper starting with the red at the top of the paper and then work down in washes of the rainbow colours (red, orange, yellow, green, blue, indigo and violet).

- If you feel like it you can then do another painting with undulating rainbow colours.

- Then you can progress to the next stage and paint a nature landscape scene in amongst the rainbow colours.

- When you have finished stand back and review your pictures asking yourself:

How do you feel now? Soothed, excited, frustrated, happy?

Were you drawn to any particular colour? If so, do you know why?

What emotion did a specific colour evoke?

If you are feeling uncomfortable in any way from this experience, ask yourself 'what is my inner wisdom trying to tell me?

Make any notes in your journal and/or make another image of the answer.

Let the feelings out however they might appear to you.

Colour can evoke many different emotions and can hold different associations for you, so just be mindful of its effect and be gentle with yourself for anything that emerges.

Colour Infusion

(For everyone)

Experiment with colour!

Each colour has a particular association to us for whatever reason. It is really interesting and liberating to experiment with different colours to express emotions.

Please note: Colour is very powerful and these exercises may have an effect on you. Observe how you feel after an exercise. You may wish to do a general picture using more colours to neutralise the effect of a specific colour.

- Lay out your paper and paints, brushes, water jar and cloth or tissue.

- Sit quietly and tune into your deeper self or do the centring process.

- Let your Self be guided into the realm of your feelings and see what emotions are present. You might be feeling angry, sad, confused, happy, ecstatic, scared, bored, tired, in love, etc.

- When you are ready, let the colour present itself to you spontaneously. You may be drawn to red or warm colours for example if you are feeling passionate, angry, alive or whatever red represents for you.

- Paint over a whole sheet of paper and experiment with the depth and tone of colour. Your image can be abstract, representational but more importantly an expression of your emotion in this moment.

- When you have finished (you may wish to do more as well), stand back and review your image.

Ask yourself why you chose that colour?

Was it an accurate representation of your emotion or did it change during the process?

How do you feel now that you have expressed that emotion or emotions?

Has the process helped you let go of that emotion or is it still present?

If you feel you are not complete, then you may wish to do more colour exercises or try a free painting of what is going on for you right now. You may also wish to make notes in your journal.

Common Colour Associations

Here are some common colour associations that I have borrowed from *The Art Therapy Sourcebook* by Cathy A. Malchiodi. Obviously any colour can have its own personal association for you and does not have to match the list below – you are free to choose – it is only a guideline:

- Red

Birth, blood, fire, emotion, warmth, love, passion, wounds, anger, heat, life.

- Orange

Fire, harvest, warmth, energy, misfortune, alienation, assertiveness, power.

- Yellow

Sun, light, warmth, wisdom, intuition, hope, expectation, energy, riches, masculinity.

- Green

Earth, fertility, vegetation, nature, growth, cycles of renewal, envy, over protectiveness, creativity.

- Blue

Sky, water, sea, heaven, spirituality, relaxation, cleansing, nourishing, calm, loyalty.

- Violet/Purple

Royalty, spirituality, wealth, authority, death, resurrection, imagination, attention, excitement, paranoia, persecution.

- Black

Darkness, emptiness, mystery, beginning, womb, unconscious, death, depression, loss.

- Brown

Fertility, soil, sorrow, roots, earth, excrement, dirt, worthlessness, new beginnings.

- White

Light, virginity, purity, moon, spirituality, creation, timelessness, dreamlike, generative, resurrection, clarity, loss, synthesis, enlightenment.

The Goddess Within

(For women)

Each Goddess exudes a certain energy which is unique to her and may resonate with our own self. The following exercise can awaken the archetypal goddess within you.

If you were a Goddess, who would you be?

- Sitting quietly, you may wish to do a relaxation process to allow yourself to come into your body.

- Read through the list of goddesses from around the world and see which one speaks to you. You may already know of the Myth or Story that is connected to the particular goddess you choose, or it may just be the name.

Some of the World's Goddesses and their meaning

(I have gathered this list from various sources and it is by no means comprehensive. There are more goddesses and more definitions to each goddess).

Greek Goddesses

Aphrodite – Goddess of love, beauty and fertility.

Ariadne (Minoan Cretan) – The pure one.

Artemis – Goddess of the wild, the hunt.

Athena – Goddess of war and crafts (and wisdom).

Circe – Magical witch (daughter of the Sun God Helios).

Daphne – Virgin huntress.

Demeter – Earth Mother, goddess of vegetation, fruitfulness and fertility.

Electra – Fire or spark.

Gaia – The Great Earth Mother.

Hecate – Goddess of the crossroads (3 directions), the moon, wise witch and death.

Hera – Lady Earth, mother goddess, home maker, protects married women.

Hestia – Goddess of the hearth.

Persephone – Goddess of fertility and queen of the underworld.

Rhea – Daughter of Gaia and Uranus.

Selene – Goddess of the Moon.

Sophia – Goddess of wisdom, heaven, the stars.

Roman Goddesses

Diana – Goddess of the wild, protector of women and girls.

Minerva – Goddess of wisdom (like Athena), war, the arts, the underworld.

Venus – Goddess of love (like Aphrodite).

Vesta – Goddess of the hearth both in the house and in the ceremonial flame.

Virginia – Constitutional change.

Celtic Goddesses

Aine – Goddess of love and fertility.

Anu, Danu, Dana – Mother Goddess.

Brigid – Goddess of healing and fertility.

Rhiannon (Welsh) – Goddess of the earth and fertility, horses, birds, and links to the Underworld.

Cybele (Phrygian) – Mother Goddess, fertility.

Don - Mother Goddess.

Arianrhod – Goddess of the sky.

Nordic Goddesses

Freya – Goddess of fertility and love.

Fjorgyn – Goddess of the earth.

Frigg – Goddess of fertility. Friday named after her. She tells no fortunes yet knows all fates.

Grid – Frost Goddess.

Idun – Goddess of spring and youth.

Sif – Goddess of the harvest.

Egyptian Goddesses

Hathor – Cow Goddess, Love, Dance, Song, Mother and Children. She nurtured the living and carried the dead to the underworld.

Isis – Mother Goddess.

Maat – Goddess of truth, justice and harmony.

Nut – Sky Goddess.

Tefnut – Goddess of moisture.

Babylonian Goddesses

Ishtar – Queen of heaven, Love and War

Babylonian Pantheon

Zarpanitu – Birth Goddess.

Sumerian Pantheon Goddesses

Ereshkigal – Queen of the underworld.

Inana – Goddess of fertility.

Ki – Earth Goddess.

Ningal – Reed Goddess.

Ninlil – Grain Goddess.

Islam Goddess

Fatima – Mother Goddess.

Indian Goddesses

Durga (aka. Kali, Uma) – Ruler of death and destruction but also motherhood.

Ganga – great River Goddess, holiness and purity.

Lakshmi – Wealth and fortune. She sits on a lotus – symbol of the womb – immortality and spiritual purity.

Maya – Miraculous power and mother of Gautama Buddha.

Parvati – Mother Goddess.

Saraswati – Sacred river goddess, watery, gives fertility and wisdom to earth.

Shakti – Force, power, energy.

Sita – Agriculture and vegetation.

Buddhist Goddesses

Aditi (Vedic) – Mother Goddess.

Tara (Buddhist) – Embodies the feminine aspect of compassion. The Essence of the goddess has 21 different forms, such as Green Tara, White Tara, etc.

Amaterasu (Shinto/Japan) – Sun Goddess.

Uzume (Shinto/Japan) – Goddess of dawn and laughter.

Kuan Yin (Chinese Buddhism) – Mercy and compassion. Helps earth people.

Kwannon (aka Kuan Yin) (Japanese Buddhism) – Mercy and compassion. Attain enlightenment. Blesses women with children. She is known as 'Lady Giver of Children' (Cotterell/Storm)

African Goddesses

Yemaya – Goddess of the ocean and mother of all.

Oshun – Goddess of the river or sweet waters.

Hawaii Goddess

Pele – Goddess of the Volcano.

Balinese Goddesses

Cili – Goddess of fertility.

Setesuyara – Goddess of the Underworld and the creator of the light and the earth (with Batara Kala).

Also refer to the Indian Hindu Goddesses above.

Christian Goddesses

Eve – Mother of all living.

Virgin Mary – Mother goddess.

Yin = Feminine.

Once you have made your choice, make an image of any aspect of the Goddess that is speaking to you. You can use any materials and take as long as you like. Really try and penetrate this Goddess energy as much as you can and see what emerges!

Stand back and review your image.

What Goddess did you chose and why?

What association do you have with this Goddess?

How do you feel this Goddess is connected to an aspect of you?

What are you trying to express through your choice of Goddess?

There is no right or wrong choice, just a potential deeper insight into your inner world.

Feel free to make any notes in your journal.

The Myth of Persephone - A Journey of Womanhood

(For women)

The myth of Persephone and the pomegranate begins when Persephone was a girl – she was also known as Kore. Innocent Kore loved to play in the meadows gathering flowers with her friends.

One day there was a tremendous noise as a big zigzag-shaped gash opened in the ground and out rode a man on a chariot pulled by black horses. His name was Hades and he was the god of the Underworld. He seized Kore and dragged her screaming down into his underground kingdom.
As the ground closed up, her cries became quieter, and all went back to normal as though nothing had happened.

The only one to hear or see anything was the old wise crone woman Hecate. She allowed the story to unfold without interfering.

Kore/Persephone's mother was called Demeter and she was the goddess of wheat and crops. She allowed everything in the world to grow and flourish. When she realised her precious daughter had disappeared, she flew into a rage and searched high and low. In her sorrow, she made all the trees, plants and crops cease to grow. She roamed the lands calling out and becoming very depressed. Everything was dead and all the people begged her to restore the land back to vegetation. But she was punishing the world for her loss.

One day as she lay exhausted against a rock with her hair all knotted and her face dirty, in a place where she was unknown, up waddled a funny looking woman. This was no ordinary woman but rather a magical, dancing, sexy woman with nipples for her eyes and a vulva for a mouth. Demeter was so shocked at this funny sight that she could not help showing a little smile. This woman, who is known as the Goddess Baubo, told her juicy rude jokes, and was as coarse and dirty as the earth itself. Demeter could not help but laugh and it became louder and deeper until her depression lifted and she continued her search once more with the help of Baubo, Hecate and the sun god Helios. They finally located Persephone and negotiated her return.

Persephone had become queen of the underworld and in some ways enjoyed her status but still wanted to return to earth. Hades loved her very much and said she could return but gave her a Pomegranate before her departure. Persephone only ate some of the seeds but this meant she would have to spend half of the year with him in the underworld and half of the year on earth.

No sooner had Persephone returned when the land was restored to its flourishing self and they all lived happily until her return to Hades.

This has also been associated with the beginning of the Seasons where Persephone returns to earth in the Spring and everything grows in Spring and Summer. She then goes back to the underworld in the Autumn and Winter when the land dies and the seeds are nourished in the dark earth.

The Goddess Baubo represents the juicy side of women when they get together and create that deep belly laugh that no man can share.

*   *   *

The story of Persephone is an archetypal story of the different stages of being a woman (or the feminine aspects within a man). The innocent child playing in the field. The dawning of consciousness or the waking up at puberty through the intellect and sexuality as portrayed by the Hades character. It may be seen as a literal 'man kidnapping an innocent girl to have his way with' but I see it as the metamorphosis of adolescence, sexuality and maturity. Then there is the life giving mother of all who is full of passion and power. The wise woman or crone who sees all but is wise enough not to interfere. And then the often left out character of Baubo who is said to be a walking vagina with breasts for eyes who wobbles and dances and sings rude songs and is the pure earthly/earthy, sexual, comedic, element that is the only one to lift Demeter out of her depression. Demeter is then able to restore the earth to creation instead of destruction and reunite with her daughter who goes on to live between the underworld and the upper world

The Main Characters

Kore: the virgin, innocent maiden.

Persephone: the transformed Kore after she returns from the underworld of Hades.

Demeter: Kore/Persephone's mother and the great Earth Mother of all.

Hecate: the wise woman or crone and Demeter's mother.

Baubo: the funny, earthy, dirty/crude, pure sexuality in all women.

Hades: ruler of the underworld. This could also represent the awakening of puberty or the unconscious part of our Self.

- Once you have read the story of Demeter, tune into any character or scene that touches you.
- Make an image representing your choice using any medium.

How do you feel about this character or scene?

What did it evoke in you?

What feelings or emotions did it bring up and why?

Write down your thoughts on the process too, if you like, in your journal.

My sister Isabella, who is an Integrative Psychotherapist, trained in Transformative Arts for Therapy and in Movement using the Tamalpa method and Biodanza Vital Development, runs wonderful workshops on these types of Myths, inspiring Women to explore aspects of themselves through art, movement and self exploration. Visit her website for more information www.lifespanpsychotherapy.co.uk.

The Core Belief Process

(For women)

This exercise is really good for identifying what we think about the bigger picture. It asks vital questions which will enhance our self knowledge and help us to gain a deeper understanding of our relationship to the Feminine.

Find a quiet place and bring your journal, some loose paper, pens, pencils and a glass of water to drink. Ask yourself the following questions, one at a time, and write your answer. Keep going until you have answered all the questions.

- What does being a woman mean to you?

- What does the Feminine mean to you?

- What makes you most angry/sad about being a woman?

- What are you most grateful for – for being a woman?

- How would you like the picture or nature of being a woman/the feminine to be in the future? How would you like it to change?

- How do we (women) move forward?

- Name one or more things you have done, achieved, received, or an insight, that celebrates you as a woman – a brag, however large or small.

- Name at least one or more things you desire. This can be material, relationship, physical, spiritual, life purpose related or to just have a fun day!

- Think of something pleasurable you can do for yourself in the next 24 hours!

- Breathe this three times into your body/being.

- Shake it out – have a dance break!

- Reflect on your answers and make notes in your journal or make an image.

Forgiveness Process

(Inspired by a specific SOURCE Process exercise called For Giving by Binnie A. Dansby)

(For everyone)

Forgiveness is a loaded word. The definition of forgiveness in the Oxford English Dictionary is 'to grant free pardon and to give up all claim on account of an offense or debt'. Many people have had difficult relationships, especially with their parents (either one or both) and yet our parents are the people who enabled our creation to take place through the love for each other and the pleasure they exchanged. There was less psychological awareness in the past, cultural conditioning still prevailed and women were supposed to just 'get on with it' quietly. It is not surprising that generations have struggled with parental relationships leaving their fragile Self in a state of perpetual grief. The inner child is constantly trying to protect the Self from re experiencing the hurt that it felt during childhood and traumatic events can almost arrest the development of the individual and leave the child unable to grow up from that point. Blame is the usual outcome.

Forgiveness, for me, is more about acceptance. For example, the difficult relationships we had in the past with our parents cannot be changed. We, however, can learn to change our story and our relationship to that story. I was very sceptical but it has certainly worked for me. As it turns out, the more I learned to forgive and accept my parents and put myself in their shoes, magic began to happen. Above all, I did not expect them to change but acknowledge them for the good they did with the knowledge and understanding they had at the time. None of us are perfect and we all try our best from where we are on the spectrum of life! So forgiveness can set you free and enhance emotional and physical wellbeing.

- Set out your art material and try not to be interrupted if possible. You may wish to do this process at different times (for your mother, for your father and for your Self) or consecutively.

- Start by doing the Take a Breath process and really allow your particular parent to come into your consciousness and into your heart. Breathe in and out rhythmically. Give them their moment in your heart space to tell you what they need the most.

Process for your Mother

- Ask yourself: What does my mother need the most right now? And let any answers come to you gently and without force. This can be emotional, physical, mental, spiritual, or anything that needs to find expression.

- When you are ready, make an image of what your mother needs the most.

Repeat this Process for your father

- Next, ask yourself: What does my father need the most? And let the answers filter to the surface in your own time. Again this can be emotional, physical, mental, spiritual, or anything that needs to find expression.

- Make an image when you are ready about what your father needs the most.

Repeat this Process for You

- Lastly, think of your young self at the age of about 5 years. Ask your little child self what she needs the most. Let your imagination wander.

- Make an image of what the little You needs the most.

Repeat this Process with the little You and your Parents together

- Bring your parents into the picture with you and let them acknowledge the little You. Allow your parents to give you a gift. Listen in and make an image of anything you receive. Be intuitive and try not to approach this from an intellectual point of view. Just let the paint, or whatever material you use, guide the process. It can be abstract, symbolic, shapes or colours, or it can represent something recognisable.

- When you have finished, take some time to reflect on your images.

What are they telling you?

How do you feel?

Remember to breathe!

If you do this exercise often, it can really help to heal the hurts of the past.

*You don't have to suddenly forgive your parents, or specific people who have hurt you but you might begin to understand them from a different point of view. Breathe and know you are loved.

Talisman & Totem

(For everyone)

A Talisman is 'Something that produces extraordinary effects, especially in averting or repelling evil; an amulet, a charm; a talisman to avert diseases' (Webster, 1913).

A Totem is 'anything which serves as a venerated or mystic symbol or emblem' (PJC)

Make an object out of any material that serves as a symbolic charm, talisman, or totem for Conception, Pregnancy, Birth, Parenthood, Loss, Baby, Dreams, Love, etc.

Conception Exercises

For Individuals and Couples

Creative Conception

(For Individuals and Couples)

Here is a wonderful process you can try if you desire conception. Conception can be a conscious event just like birth or raising a child. Just because we assume that we just 'get pregnant' it does not mean we are not able to creatively invite it into our lives.

We must remember that it takes two people to conceive a baby; it is not just the woman. Conception is not an intellectual process that you can fit into your scheduled diaries or put on your 'to do' list. Make time for your conception and honour the creative process that it is without trying to make it happen; otherwise you will create unnecessary stress and anxiety.

These exercises can be done alone or with your partner. This is a great opportunity to involve your partner into the 'self exploratory' arena of pregnancy, and not just doing the fun stuff. You may wish to do this alone first so you can express your authentic feelings just in case you edit them or gloss over your true feelings if you do it with your partner (I'm not saying you will and it depends on your relationship and what you feel is best).

Doing this exercise by yourself:

- Set out some of your art materials ready for your spontaneous choice.

- Begin with the centring process and/or some deep breathing. Sit in a comfortable place, free from interruptions, preferably with your eyes closed if this feels ok.

- Gently lay one hand on your belly and the other hand on your pubic bone/genitals.

- Stay like this for a while, tuning into where your hands are and see if any thoughts, feeling, or images emerge.

- Is there anything you need to express right now?

- Is there anything you wish to forgive yourself for, like feeling or thinking a certain way about your body; for any behaviour, or for feeling that you are/were wrong in any way?

+ Ask your inner child if she is ok with you conceiving a baby? Does she have something to say? Reassure her that everything is taken care of and she will still be number one.

+ What do you think about babies, being a mother, being a woman, your body, your relationship, men and the masculine, the higher powers?

Once you have mulled over these questions, see which art materials you gravitate towards and make an image or a few images. Remember, there is no right or wrong, so no judgement about what emerges from this exercise.

You may also wish to write freely in your journal about thoughts, feelings or images that arose.

In doing these exercises over time you will begin to uncover how you feel about having a baby – or having another baby.

Doing this exercise with your partner:

You can begin the same way with one of the relaxation processes if you wish and maybe even sit opposite each other holding hands. See if you can breathe together. This will also stimulate even deeper intimacy.

When you feel ready, place your own hands on your own belly and genitals. This can also help men to connect to their sexuality and innocence and their desire to procreate. Placing his hand on his belly can help him connect to his life force. A man also has a history that needs acknowledgement. He may have experienced emotional, physical or even sexual abuse, a traumatic birth, low self esteem and not see himself as the powerful life creator that he is, or doubt his ability to be a father to another human being and so on.

Revel in this time together and mull over some of the questions below. Try not to strain your brain but just let the thoughts come and go and just be aware of thoughts or images that come to the surface as you sit together in stillness. Also, try not to feel pressured to think up an image, this is supposed to be relaxing, insightful and maybe even fun.

Here are some interesting questions you may wish to contemplate, without judgement. You can either write about or makes images, collages, sculptures or anything that you feel inspired to create:

+ Do you think you have to be married in order to conceive a baby?

136

- Do you think you have to have a certain income or financial status before you conceive a baby?

- Do you think you have to be a certain age to have children? Do you think you are too young or too old or just not ready?

- Is there anything holding you back?

- Do you want to conceive a baby because all of your friends are having children?

- Are there any fertility issues that you are aware of?

- Do you feel impatient? (There is divine timing with conception and even birth).

There is a school of thought that suggests the unborn child chooses her parents, culture and set of circumstances that she is born into, and our job is to remain open and joyful in the process.

Exercises for Couples: Celebrating *Her* Body

Here is a ritual you can do with your partner that deepens intimacy and adds fun into the co creation process. This is not necessarily about ending in intercourse, so try not to feel pressured, but purely about appreciating the body and the role of a woman's genitals and reproductive capacity. It is also a good chance for a woman to learn to overcome any shame she may have in that area and to Receive.

- Body ritual for the woman: Celebrate your Divine Source (genitals, vagina, yoni, pussy) by allowing your partner to pay homage to your central area of creation (your genital area). Worship her like a goddess.

- Find a comfortable place that is free from distractions and feels safe and nurturing. This is important for total relaxation, safety and enjoyment.

- You may wish to light candles, put on sensual music, wear something that makes you feel good i.e. something silky and loose or nothing at all but make sure you are warm, comfortable and ready to be honoured.

- You may wish to decorate your pubic bone area with sequins or in a way that pleases you.

- Let your partner look at your genitals and say nice things to her, for instance how beautiful she looks. Receive your partner's compliments.

- Partner: Tease her with a feather, fur or something sensual of your choice.

- Massage her body with sacred essential oils.

- Draw, paint or sculpt her Divine Source. You can both do this part.

- If you want to swap and honour your partner, it is possible but not compulsory.

If possible... just have FUN!

Affirmations you can both use:

- I am Innocent.

- My body is Innocent.

- I innocently make love with my partner in joyous union, as an expression of love.

- I am open to receive a child into my life.

- I trust my body.

- I love my body.

- I am a Creatrix – a co-creator.

*You may wish to try any Exercise in the next chapters on Pregnancy, Birth, Loss, or the General Self Development Exercises. Any exercise that feels right for you, and could help free the way towards conception, is recommended.

Pregnancy Exercises

For Pregnant Women and Partners

The Magic Question

(For pregnant women and partners)

This is a very important question because any pregnant woman (and her partner) has a myriad of thoughts, feelings, hopes, fears, joys, and expectations surrounding her pregnancy.

Set out a selection of different art materials, whatever you have.

- Find time when you won't be disturbed.

- Start with one of the relaxation processes to allow yourself to journey within.

- When you have finished the relaxation exercise, ask yourself this question:

How do I feel about having a baby?

Do not judge the answers or images that arise, let them all come and wash over you.

Make an image on any one of your thoughts or feelings. You can also write about them in your journal, either stream of consciousness style, or just notes.

Your Fantasy Birth

(For pregnant women)

What 'mood' would you like for your birth? This is a great question to ask yourself because it takes you away from a specific or desired 'birth outcome'. You and your supporters can aim to maintain this envisioned birth mood whatever the outcome.

Sit or lie down wherever you feel most comfortable and inspired. Feel your body sink into the support that is taking your weight. Take a few deep breaths and you may wish to make a noise on the out breath to really let out any tension. Gently remind yourself that this is your special time to go within and that all you wish to express and feel is welcome. You have permission to create in your mind anything that you feel would support your birthing.

Try and visualise your birth, get in touch with the mood. Ask yourself some questions:

- What would I like my labour and birth to look like?

- Where would I feel most comfortable to give birth?

- What kind of sounds or music would support me?

- What sort of lighting would support me?

- Who would I like present at my birth?

- What is the overall feeling I would like to experience?

- What could I do or overcome in order to create this mood?

Birth is messy, dirty, earthy, it asks for a total surrendering of control, a surrendering of the mind. Delve into the underworld of your subconscious and release anything that may hold you back so you can bring forth your baby to this world with greater ease.

'The dark and bloody Goddesses of transformation are always healers. They direct us to those forbidden inner territories where our blocked energies have been locked up and bolted down for years. The tension experienced in the pre-menstrual phase is the battle between the free spirit of our potential and the tranquillized persona of passivity we are expected to present to the world' (Sunflower, Chapter 7, p163, in Voices of the Goddess, a Chorus of Sibyls, edited by Caitlin Matthews, 1990).

'The pre-menstrual phase can be a time when feelings, especially aggressive, angry ones, involutes into depression because we as women are not allowed to become the raging lioness, the wild beast that is part of us'. (P161-2)

Although these quotes refer to the menstrual phase they conjure the deeper truth that women often experience in life, especially during pregnancy and birth. I love the image of a raging lioness giving birth to the next generation in all her power and glory!

- Once you have delved into your fantasy world and created a desired mood in your imagination, take art materials, if this feels pleasurable, and make some art. It can be abstract or realistic, two or three dimensional, and in any media.

Mirror rorriM

(For women, especially pregnant women)

+ Look in the mirror and repeat as often as you wish: 'I love you... (Your name)'. It is important to feel as much self love and acceptance as possible as the baby grows inside your body. You are not only giving birth to your baby but to a new you – whether it is your first baby or your fifth! Each time, you too are born again.

+ The Vagina, or Divine Source, is the most intimate piece of your anatomy and is the opening through which your baby will come into this world. The second mirror exercise invites you to get to know and build a positive relationship with your precious Divine Source.

+ So with your hand mirror, find a quiet, comfortable place, free from distractions or interruptions where you can recline. You may wish to find lovely cushions to make yourself more comfortable. Maybe light a candle or burn some sensual incense and make sure you have good lighting so you can see your genitals. Have a good look! You may wish to follow on to the exercise on Vagina Art in the next section.

+ In the third Mirror exercise, find the part of your body that you most dislike and say to it: 'I love you'. 'You are perfect'. Begin to feel the genuine acceptance of that body part because you are delicious exactly as you are.

Divine Source/Yoni/Vagina/Cunt/Pussy Art You Name Her!

(For pregnant women or any woman wishing to celebrate her Divine Source)

Celebrate your precious Divine Source by making art in her honour. This can be a fun mixed media extravaganza!

Use fabric, glitter, sequins, ribbon or anything you can find that inspires you. You will probably need glue, scissors and maybe even a needle and thread. You can use either paper, card (even a cardboard box!) or a canvas (these can be purchased very cheaply in the most random places... I've bought perfectly adequate ones in the 99p shop)!

- Before you begin, take a moment to tune into your body and notice how it is feeling. What thoughts or feelings are bubbling under the surface?

- Excitement, shame, feeling naughty, disgusted, empowered?

- Do not judge them, just make a note.

- You may wish to jot any of these feelings down in your journal or draw a quick spontaneous picture.

- When you feel ready, you can simply experiment. Have fun, go wild, release any shame, and revel in your most precious anatomical area! You can create an image from memory, a fictional one or you can get the mirror out if you prefer. The point is to have fun creating the essence of this piece of anatomy. There is no right or wrong!

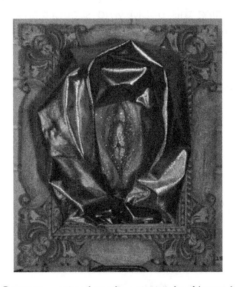

My Divine Source – mixed media painting by Alexandra Florschutz

The Sensual Wonders of Water

(For pregnant women)

If you enjoy water, having a bath can be a wonderful and sensual experience. If you do not have a bath then maybe a friend would let you borrow theirs. Keep the water close to your body temperature, under 100 degrees Fahrenheit. If the water is too hot you may overheat which raises your heartbeat. Drink plenty of water. A water birthing pool is another option which has a built-in temperature regulator. It is a great way to ease tired muscles.

Tune into your baby. Is there anything you want to ask her? Your baby is listening. Ask your baby what she needs. Tell her a story.

Nurturing network

(For pregnant women and partners)

Seek out a network of people – whether pregnant or already parents (depending on where you are when reading this book) who support and believe that birth is easy, natural and normal. It is important to connect to like-minded people who can offer a listening ear, cuddles and a good cup of tea!

I will also have a facility on my website www.theartofbirth.co.uk to offer counselling via email or Skype.

The Secret Key to your Symptoms

(For pregnant women)

Louise L. Hay and others believe that our thoughts about ourselves and about life create illness and symptoms in our physical body. In this light, it is worth looking at our pregnancy symptoms and see what wisdom they hold. Pregnancy can certainly bring on certain ailments but it is worth looking at the psychological roots behind the symptom.

- Make time and tune into materials that you are attracted to.

- Sitting quietly in a safe place, begin by doing a relaxation process.

- Ask yourself: What is this symptom trying to tell me?

- Whatever images or words filter to the surface just allow them to flow without judgement.

- You may wish to write about your symptom too. For example, sickness, which is a very common symptom. What does it mean to you?

Ask yourself perhaps: What do I not wish to digest? What am I rejecting? Fear of the new? Naturally, it may just be the way in which the baby is positioned or any reason, but your symptom could be the key to your health.

Your Previous Birth Story/Stories

(For women of all ages, pregnant women)

It is really helpful to write, draw, paint, sculpt your birth story or stories. Expressing all the emotions that surround any birth story, can really help to free the way for the next birth. Some births can be very traumatic and linger for many years while others, even if they were more straightforward, might still benefit from processing.

- Set out all art materials that you might want to use.

- Sit quietly and, if you feel like it, do a relaxation process and tune into your story.

- Make an image of your birth story or a series of images. These images are pictorial manifestations of suppressed memories and are better released than held in your unconscious. Try not to judge it in any way whatever comes up.

You are innocent and whatever you express is welcome!

Make notes in your journal if you feel like it.

Your Family

(For pregnant women and parents)

It is really helpful to tune into how your new baby's arrival will fit into the existing family. If you have other children, how does it feel to be having another child? Was this child planned or a surprise? Is it your second child or do you have several? Do you have boys or girls and if so, do you have a preference for the next child?

+ Start this process by setting up your art materials.

+ Sit or lie quietly, uninterrupted – if possible – and tune into your family

+ Consider the questions above and see what surfaces.

+ Make an image, collage, drawing, or write in your journal.

Inner Guide Meditation

(For pregnant women – and everyone)

+ Set out your art materials, journal, clay or anything you want to work with.

This guided Visualisation evokes a powerful person/being, a symbol of strength that you can manifest as your inner guide and support which you can call upon any time.

Position yourself as comfortably as you can on your chair
Shifting your weight so that your body can feel fully supported
Rest your open hands on your lap
Feel your feet on the floor
Close your eyes if this feels comfortable
Take some deep, full cleansing breaths
Just let everything fall away
Knowing that you are safe and all is taken care of right now

And again, breathe in
And this time see if you can send the warm energy of the breath to any part of your body that is tense or sore or tight
And release the tension with the exhale and breathe it out

And any unwelcome thoughts that come to mind, those too can be sent out with the breath, released with the exhale.

Now, imagine yourself outdoors on a calm, sunny day
Find yourself in a clearing in a wood
Notice the smells and sounds
And you feel very safe

You see a path that leads up through the woods
Walking slowly

Feeling the texture of the ground beneath your feet
Whether it is sand or pine needles or grass
And the warm air on your skin

Then you come to a clearing
There is a fire in the middle
On the far side of the fire is a beautiful wise woman, as ancient as time but as youthful as the dawn
She is your wise inner guide
She is weaving cloth out of star beams
She waits quietly

Place a log on the fire
Sparks dance and crackle
The wise woman beckons to you
You go and sit next to her
What is she like?
What would you like to know?

When you are ready, ask her a question – whatever springs to mind in the moment
Take your time and listen for the answer

Rest a while
Then thank your wise inner guide
Your wise inner guide embraces you
When you are ready to leave she gives you a gift in memory of your meeting

Walking slowly and calmly out of the clearing
And down the path
Feeling the forest under your feet, the smell, the temperature
You come to the first clearing

And once again, feel yourself sitting in your chair, breathing in and out
Very gently and with soft eyes, let yourself come back into the room
Whenever you are ready
Open your eyes

- You may wish to write in your journal, draw a picture or make something that represents your journey to your wise inner guide.

- You may wish to create a mixed media Talisman that represents your inner guide.

Free Painting

(For pregnant women and partners)

Set out a selection of your art materials. It is useful to have as many as you can so you are free to be spontaneous and choose what you desire in the moment.

- Start this exercise by doing a relaxation process to tune into your body and release your creativity.

- Make an image for 20 to 30 minutes about anything you desire or you can ask yourself the following:

- How am I feeling?

- Where am I at – at this moment in time?

- What is rising up and wanting to be expressed?

- What is my baby trying to communicate to me?

- How do I feel about being a mother/father?

When you have finished, stand back and observe your picture and see what is going on in it.

Reflect on how it makes you feel and what response you are having to your picture.

What emotions are present?

What effect are the colours having on you?

What do the different colours mean to you (what do they symbolically represent)?

What do the shapes represent?

What does the scene represent or what is it about?

If you like, make notes in your journal.

A Breath of Fresh Air

(For pregnancy and everyone)

Breathing is good! Remember to breathe fully as the breath releases stress.

A Play Date with your Self

(For women and especially for conception, pregnancy and motherhood)

At least once a week, schedule a play date with yourself. This can be anything from a walk in nature (always a good idea) to a trip to see your favourite film, a manicure or pedicure, a massage, _____fill in the blank!

The only requirement is that it is FUN and PLEASURABLE!

I, ..., pleasurably commit to ....this week.

Signed with Pleasure:... ☺

Exploring the Notion of the Feminine

(For women and especially for conception, pregnancy and motherhood)

Set out a selection of your art materials.

- Start this exercise by doing a relaxation process to tune into your body and allow you to release your creativity.

- While you are doing the relaxation process, gently ask yourself the following questions:

- What does being a Woman mean to me?

- What does the Feminine mean to me?

When you are ready, open your eyes and choose any art materials that you are drawn to. I would recommend paint but you are free to choose.

- Make an image for about 20 to 30 minutes (again this can be as long or short as you are able to manage depending on your time or pleasure).

When you have finished, stand back and observe your picture and see what is going on in it.

Reflect on how it makes you feel and what response you are having to your picture.

What emotions are present?

What effect are the colours having on you?

What do the different colours mean to you (what do they symbolically represent)?

What do the shapes represent?

What does the scene represent?

If you like, make notes in your journal.

Life after a Caesarean

The Possibility of a Vaginal Birth after Caesarean (VBAC)

(For pregnant and non pregnant women)

*You can also do any of the General Exercises or choose ones that feel relevant to you.

There are so many different views on pregnancy – whether to have this, that or the other treatment, procedure, medicine, surgery. What we think is right, wrong, acceptable or unacceptable is a very personal opinion. Many women have expressed some very mixed feelings after having experienced an emergency caesarean. On the one hand, in the case of elected caesareans, some women feel like they are in control of the birth and don't have to face the trauma of giving birth vaginally. They feel empowered by this choice. And on the other hand, there are women who would feel very disappointed and shocked if they had an emergency caesarean because it did not go according to their plan. Knowing that your birth was just right exactly the way it was is the first step to healing your experience. It is better to have a healthy baby and mother than to cling to the ideal of a 'natural vaginal birth', or any other desired outcome.

It can, however, be very liberating to explore the experience and to release any feelings attached to the outcome. Once you have expressed these feelings, such as disappointment, anger, sadness, or even relief, gratitude and joy, it is then possible to look at what might be done differently in future pregnancies. This can also apply to a traumatic vaginal birth. It is helpful to process any feelings even if you are not planning to have any more children.

Firstly, you must know that your birth was just right and you did really well!

Secondly, in hindsight, did you learn anything from your experience? Was there anything you might do differently next time?

I know many women who were so shocked at the way they were treated that they actively sought ways of healing their experience and managed to turn around the next birth in a very positive way.

It is possible to have a vaginal birth after a caesarean (vbac) and it can be helpful to process the first experience in order to prepare for the next birth. If you decide to have an elected caesarean for your next birth, you can still create a positive experience for yourself and your baby.

+ First of all set out your art materials.

+ Begin this process by doing a relaxation exercise.

+ Remember to be very gentle with yourself and try and refrain from any judgement. Just let any emotion come to the surface. Help yourself to some art materials which you feel drawn to and ask yourself: How am I feeling about this experience? What do I need to express? I am safe and innocent and have done everything exactly right.

+ Make an image or series of images of whatever comes up. It is often good to do some spontaneous 'stream of consciousness' paintings as this taps into the emotion.

Review the images. What can you see?

Are there any specific symbols?

Have you used any particular colours?

What do these colours symbolise to you?

How do you feel after doing this exercise?

Make notes of your process in your journal as this can be useful to look back on and build up a deeper picture of your experience.

Pregnancy Loss

Pregnancy Loss

Miscarriage, including failed in vitro fertilization, molar pregnancy, ectopic pregnancy, loss in multiple-gestation pregnancy, abortion and stillbirth

(For women. This exercise can also support fathers who might wish to make images on their experiences of losing a child).

Pregnancy loss is a legitimate loss albeit often an 'invisible' one. Grief work may be essential as this loss can evoke a variety of strong emotions such as immense guilt, depression, feeling out of control, paralysed, etc. The guilt can come from what we feel went wrong, or from the thought that our body was in some way dysfunctional. The depth of grief is incomparable. Pregnancy loss is often much worse than losing, for example, a living relative because there is a combination of the loss of something that has been longed for, with the feelings about how the woman's body has somehow failed in its basic biological function to have a baby. These unhelpful feelings need to be released as soon as possible so that new feelings, such as gentleness, self-compassion, love, support, understanding, innocence and eventually peace, can flow in knowing that our body did the best it could.

Artist Marion Flanary expressed how she felt in a very clear way, 'Miscarriage is a ripping away — of excitement, of dreams, of joy. A senseless emptiness remains, accompanied by profound grief.' (Cited in Seftel, L., 2006)

Frida Kahlo also painted images of her miscarriages in graphic detail which was her way of being able to process the immense feelings she experienced. We need to break the silence of pregnancy loss and learn to validate our experience with the depth of understanding it deserves.

There is also the question of different religious beliefs and how these regard an unborn child. I do not wish to pass any judgement on any belief system, whether the foetus is or is not a human being, but suggest that you (and your partner) process your feelings in a way that suits you.

- First set out your selection of art materials.

- Begin this process by doing a relaxation exercise and tune into the time of your loss, knowing that you are innocent and loved.

- Let any images come to the surface and remember to breathe fully and lovingly. Even though your pregnancy loss is essentially invisible to the physical outside world, you can represent it in any way that feels right. This can be representational, abstract, symbolic or a complete mess to purge those wild feelings. When you are ready, select your desired art materials and make an image or series of images. If words come to mind, you can also write them in your journal or on your image.

For Mothers and Fathers/Partners

+ Tell your story to a friend, counsellor, or group. Find or start a support group (for either women or men or maybe even mixed).

+ Write poetry about your experience, write a letter to your child, write a story.

+ Name your lost child, perform a burial ritual, or a symbolic burial (if there is nothing physical to bury) plant a tree, make a coffin, or one which the family can decorate, create a ritual, create a sacred space or an altar/shrine.

+ Draw, paint, collage, sculpt or make a Mandala.

+ Movement. Choose your favourite music and stand still with your feet feeling the ground beneath you. Find that place of stillness. When you feel ready, gently begin to move in whatever way you like. Feel the music wash over you. Express your feelings in the movement. Move around, stamp, roll on the floor, make noise, anything which will allow you to release your feelings through your body and voice.

+ Once again, honour your own body which had to go through an unpleasant experience and trauma. You may wish to go for a walk in nature, have a massage, a soothing bath with some essential oils, rub some special oil or lotion into your body lovingly as you soothe and caress it. Your partner can also do this for you if this feels right. In fact, any form of pleasurable self care is recommended. And Love yourself.

Pregnancy Loss

Abortion

(For women)

This exercise may support you to release any emotions still buried from your abortion. It can also be a self-soothing time for you to be creative and connect to your experience in a positive way.

- First set out your selection of art materials.

- Begin this process by doing a relaxation exercise and tune into the time of your abortion. Please do not judge yourself in any way and know that the decision you made was right for you at the time. Or notice if any judgements do come to the surface.

- Let any images come to the surface and remember to breathe fully and lovingly. When you are ready select your desired art materials and make an image or series of images. If words come to mind, you can also write them in your journal or on your image.

- One way of honouring your abortion, if you were unable to perform a ritual at the time, is to perform an imaginary ceremony. Once you have done the relaxation exercise and tuned into the event, thank the soul for coming to you and explain that the time was too soon or the circumstances were not right. You may light a candle, burn some incense or say a prayer of acknowledgement. You may wish to give the foetus or 'group of cells' a name. You may wish to plant a tree, shrub or plant in the garden in its honour. Anything that can build a positive relationship between yourself and the event will be really healing.

- You may wish to paint, write, draw or make an image/images of your feelings. Then find a cardboard box which you could decorate. Once you have put your images inside the box, burn or 'cremate' it on a fire to release your feelings and thus transform them by sending them back to the earth.

- You can also honour your own body which had to go through an unpleasant operation with i.e. a massage, a soothing bath with some essential oils, rub some special oil or lotion into your body lovingly as you soothe and caress it. In fact any form of pleasurable self care is recommended. And Love yourself.

Create an Art of Birth Group

Why not create a peer-run Art of Birth group in your community? Set a time each week to meet for two hours, perhaps in someone's house, to be creative. It is important to establish some simple boundaries.

It is really helpful to agree that what is said or made within the group stays confidential.

When you make an image, try not to interpret or analyse it for the person who made it but allow them to tell the group what it is about – if they choose.

Judgements can be both positive and negative. For example if you 'praise' a person's image, you are making a judgement and the whole idea about expressive art is that it is not about good or bad art. It is about your expression not how well you have done. Just bear this in mind.

You may inspire, be appreciated and, fundamentally, you must feel supported.

- Once everyone has arrived and had a drink, begin with a centring process.
- You may wish to run the group either as a total free expressive art group, or work through the series of themes offered on the next page.

Keep a folder of your work in a safe place and don't feel you have to show your creations to anyone if you don't want to because art-work always invites comments!

Have an inspiring time...

Themes for Art Making

(For pregnant women, partners, everyone)

Here are some themes you may wish to explore creatively, especially if you run an Art of Birth group. They can be helpful guidelines and nudge us into thinking about our life and the messages we have received which may influence the birth of our baby.

At the beginning of a session, just ask one of the questions below and let it sit with you for a while. Once it has resonated with you and you start receiving ideas or images you can start. If nothing is coming up for you, you may wish to ask yourself if this question has a particular colour or shape. You can then work with this colour or shape and something else may develop. Any way is fine and remember not to judge yourself for anything. You will get different messages on different days so don't let it put you off if some days your mind or creativity goes blank. It may mean you need a rest or some self-care and pleasure.

What was your Birth like? This can be the story that was given to you or a 'feeling' of what it might have been like.

What were the first few months after birth like for you? Were you breastfed, was there a positive attachment between you and your mother, were your parents together?

What was your childhood like – both your story and your inherited story?

What was puberty like for you? What were the messages about female cycles, body image, sexuality, being a girl or being a boy?

What was the message given to you about being a Woman?

What was the message given to you about being a Man?

What do you think about your body?

What was/is the message you have received about Birth?

How do you feel about your family (parents, siblings, aunts, uncles, grandparents)?

Is there anything in your life which you are trying to 'forget' or 'blot out'? This can be a good time to 'express' it in a creative way.

What is your relationship like with your partner?

How do you feel about being pregnant?

How do you feel about your partner having a baby/being a father/being a parent?

How do you feel about the baby growing inside your body?

How do you feel about your children (if you have any)?

What do you most need to express right now?

What do you think about God, the Goddess, Higher Power, Source, etc?

What do you think about Sex?

Mess – What is your relationship to mess?

How would you like to birth your baby?

Positive Birth Stories

Lila's Births with Ari and Ratih

I would like to introduce this chapter with the story of my sister-in-law Lila who lives in rural Bali in a small village near Ubud. She had two very different births and her story is inspiring. Her first birth was in hospital and she describes it as a 'traumatic experience' which nearly put her off having more children. Even though Bali has this wonderful natural, child centred legacy, it is striking to see how this has changed over time due to the influence of western medicine. Her birth was long and unsupported. She experienced every intervention available and was scared, in pain and remained in shock for some time after. Breastfeeding was difficult and her baby, Ari, was unsettled and distressed. Lila said she found it hard to bond with Ari and knew it was due to her having a difficult birth.

When she became pregnant with her second child she was determined to have a better experience. She had heard about a local natural birth clinic and decided to inquire. The Bumi Sehat Clinic in Ubud, run by world renowned Robin Lim, offers free maternity care for Balinese women and promotes the belief that birth can be easy and natural. Lila had acupuncture and talked to inspiring women at the clinic and this helped her to engage with her pregnancy in a different way.

Her labour was very short. She birthed in a pool filled with flower petals, while a small group of gentle yet powerful women surrounded the pool and sang soothing songs. She said she felt relaxed and safe and her baby was born easily. Breastfeeding was easy and long lasting unlike with her first child. The contrast between the two births has had an interesting impact on her children. The second child slept easily, is more relaxed, happy and contented and attached to the mother without any problem. The first child struggles with her relationship to her mother and has always been much more unsettled. Is this a coincidence? There is too much evidence to suggest otherwise and Lila is convinced it is due to her contrasting birth experiences.

*The birth stories that follow are original transcripts as I felt it was more powerful to read the author's own version and to 'hear' their voice.

Zephyr's Birth by Roma Norris (in the UK)

Describe your pregnancy and how you prepared for your birth?

I was really shocked to find out I was pregnant. My hormones had been all over the place after a severe kidney infection and it had affected my periods and confused me. My relationship with my boyfriend Jamie was not ideal, although we had been together for five years and talked about having children some day in the future. I wasn't even sure if I should keep the baby, although deep down I knew I would. Confused, shocked and scared, I went to see a wonderful therapist for guidance and received an affirming experience where I connected with the angelic realm and found a resounding YES to the baby. I was moved by seeing SO many angels and felt really supported from then onwards.

Nausea soon set in and I quickly became allergic to the city I had adored living in. The crowds, the smells, the fried chicken and wireless internet. It jarred my entire being and drove us out of the flat we had only just moved into. The nausea cleared around fifteen weeks, but my kidneys became very sore due to the pregnancy. I was really unwell for most of the first trimester, often staying in bed feeling miserable. We decided to go and stay with Jamie's mother for a few months while we found somewhere to settle, but this only resulted in a massive blow up after a few days, where she screamed at me and we realised she was very resentful towards me for all kinds of reasons. So there we were, homeless, estranged from family, rocky in our relationship and I was unwell. I remember having contractions on the day we left Jamie's mother, probably from the stress of it all.

Thankfully, a pregnant friend and her partner took us in. It was so supportive to be going through the process with them and supporting each other, although we were emotionally, financially and (me) physically a disaster! Moira and I did yoga together each morning and I would usually crawl back to bed afterwards. It was lovely to be able to cook for each other and chat about our hopes and ideas for our babies.

At seven months pregnant I was on a bus, reading, when a woman literally flew into me and landed my bump with her entire body weight! Jamie saw me turn green and hauled me off the bus in time for me to vomit on the street. We went to the hospital and they diagnosed a broken rib, but thankfully the baby was fine. From then on I was in agony, with the growing baby pushing against my rib. It was virtually impossible to sleep and at one point I became so sleep deprived that I was convinced my baby was kicking my rib on purpose, to hurt me!

We eventually found somewhere to live in the countryside, just in time for our friends to have the space to have their baby! We signed up with a well known Independent Midwife, who lived locally and agreed that we would just pay her as and when we could – even if this took years.

Were you creative during pregnancy – if so what did you do?

Shortly after we moved I discovered a woman offering weekly Birth Art Café sessions, which were amazing! Jamie and I usually went together and it gave us an opportunity to connect with our pregnancy and express our fears through artwork. I made some good friends there and continued to go for a year after Zephyr was born. We collected the artwork we made each week, which had given us so many insights, and made a beautiful birth altar in our house.

Describe your birth experience.

I had a really lazy couple of days where I just wanted to sleep all the time, no wild nesting for me! The next day, at forty weeks plus nine days, I felt light cramps coming every twenty minutes or so. I didn't think much of them at first and dismissed them as something that might go on for days. I checked in with my birth entourage – my midwife, my friend Binnie Dansby, who is an educator, philosopher and author and my friend Becca, who was a student midwife at the time. Binnie simply said "great, you're in labour Darlin'" and that was when it dawned on me. I had a bath in the afternoon, mooched around, ate a lovely meal and decided to go back to sleep.

Around 7pm I was awoken by a 'proper' contraction, which jolted me from sleep so dramatically that I momentarily panicked. Luckily, just at that moment, a gorgeous massage therapist called Sophie Shenstone arrived at our house to give me a massage we had booked a while ago in case I was still pregnant! It was totally blissful and put me in such a relaxed, joyful mood. Sophie knew exactly where to hold while I was contracting and it felt great. She left around 9pm, just as Binnie arrived! I sat with Binnie in the kitchen, eating ice lollies for a bit and then we went upstairs to the room we had prepared for birth. We had our gorgeous altar decorated with all our birth art and the most amazing abundance of huge white roses.

Contractions started to become really intense and I stayed on my hands and knees and rolled forward onto a ball with each one. My friend Becca arrived. My waters went, which took me by surprise. We called the midwife shortly afterwards and she arrived at 11pm. I felt pretty relaxed, able to cope and blissed-out during the first stage of labour.

Around 1am, contractions were coming hard and fast and I enquired about whether I could go in the pool yet. What I had not realised is that our boiler had packed up and people were frantically boiling pans and kettles. Two more friends had arrived, but remained very much in the background. Eventually the pool was ready and it was such a relief to get in there. Contractions were feeling much harder to deal with now and I was making a noise somewhere between a yell and a really loud Ommmm. At this point I started to doubt myself and became paranoid that my midwife thought I needed to go to hospital for some reason. In hindsight, I was just in transition and needed some heavy reassurance. After two hours in the pool, my baby was very close and I felt his head just inside my vagina. I looked around in astonishment at my supporters, exclaiming "the head! The head!"

But somehow I had allowed doubt to creep in and the fear made the experience suddenly painful and overwhelming. My midwife suggested I get out of the pool and she could try a manoeuvre that entailed me lying on my back and pulling my feet to my chest; pushing hard with each contraction. This was sheer agony and after screaming through a few contractions I refused to go on and turned back onto my knees. I hung my arms around Jamie's neck and it felt really good to have him to pull against as I pushed our baby out. Our midwife passed him through my legs and into my hands and he cried for quite a long time. The labour had been quite hard going for both of us; his head was very moulded and his eye was bruised and some of my first words to Zephyr were an apology that the birth had taken so long. It was so beautiful to receive him and put him straight to my chest; it completed something within me that had been missing since my own birth. We were surrounded by friends in our lovely home as dawn broke and our beautiful son had his first feed.

What would you say helped you to have your birth outcome?

I did a *lot* of therapy of all kinds while I was pregnant! I don't think this is necessarily essential for everyone, but I personally felt I had a huge leap to make before I could be entrusted with a precious being… and I only had nine months to prepare! I read a *lot* of books, did weekly couples therapy to work on our relationship, and did Emotional Freedom Technique to rewrite my experience of my own birth in order that I wouldn't recreate a premature birth. I did sessions of SOURCE Breathwork, which helped me to get in touch with my own experiences of being in the womb and being born and helped me heal them so that they wouldn't impact on my own experience. Because I was also physically unwell, I saw a homeopath, naturopath and a reflexologist regularly. I always say you can't just plan a homebirth; you have to prepare for it. For me, there was a lot that needed to be done to clear the beliefs and fears that would have become obstacles to a positive birth.

Your 'top tip' for a more pleasurable birth.

Do the work you need to do on yourself. Our fears around birth can take over when we are in the altered state of consciousness that labour brings. It is essential to really get to the root of and clear these limiting thoughts, not just suppress them. When women are truly approaching birth from the right space, they tend to make choices that will support them.

Birth of Cahya by Jelila (in Bali)

The Yoga of Motherhood
What it means to have a child – and what an opportunity for growth it is!

Cahya looks up at me with steely blue, quizzical eyes, and starts to suckle for the first time. She is so beautiful, a tiny little square body, all folded up, like an oven-ready chicken at the supermarket. Her tiny feet are blue – the blood is just starting to course through her body with her first breaths, and her face is becoming pink. Finally, we are together, after nine months of waiting.

These are the first precious moments of our daughter Cahya, and perhaps the most precious moment of my life, too.

Nothing can describe the love that a mother has for her child; nothing can surpass it or even begin to tell you its depth and power. It is only since giving birth myself that I have really realised how much my own mother loves me, and also, what a gift a mother is.

It was a strange birth, especially by Balinese standards (where women are shunted on a production line, pumped with drugs, routinely cut open, and this miraculous and sacred process is really not allowed to unfold naturally at all.) We decided to have a home birth in our place at Tebesaya, Ubud. We were staying in a great, open plan hall of a house, eight sided, perfect Feng Shui. Big beanbags, lots of space, private and quiet, ideal for a birth, really.

(I do find it bizarre that women are expected to give birth in certain places like hospitals. Narrow, high, single iron hospital beds! I looked at them and was like, 'yes and where am I supposed to give birth?' And, as for the idea of moving from the birth suite to another 'delivery room' for the final birth – well that is completely preposterous! I have never heard of such a ludicrous idea. It's rather like suggesting that during sex, you move to a different room for orgasm – not exactly adding flow to the process is it?)

Anyway, my husband Putu, in his usual extraordinary way, agreed to my home birth plans, which were really 'luar biasa' ('far out') by Balinese standards, where everyone just goes to hospital. He set himself to work, building a birthing pool from bamboo and tarpaulin (it worked very well and even allowed the necessary and mythical task of 'boiling lots of water' for a birth, which was nice). Shortly before the birth he arrived proudly with the ceremonial coconut container and small offerings that would be used for the 'ari ari' or afterbirth.

The Balinese believe in a very strong link between the afterbirth and the baby. They believe the afterbirth contains the 'little sister' of the baby – something like the 'four humours' from ancient English medieval beliefs, actually – air, earth, fire and water. The afterbirth is placed in the coconut and buried by the front door. Flower offerings are placed there for a month after the birth and then a stone is put on top of the space. Every time the child leaves the house, earth is touched near the stone and touched to the child's forehead. In this way she 'takes leave' of her little sister.

Weaving this local belief into our birth story was easy for me – Putu had the main adjusting to do, as he felt a lot of responsibility for me and was worried that something might go wrong with what was for him and his culture, quite an outlandish plan.

Our midwife, Debra, arrived from America some days before the birth. Practical and down to earth, she inspired confidence and was a great birth partner. (We also had a link arranged to the best local obstetrician, and transport ready – just in case).

Birth, it seems funny to need to say it, is 'a girl thing'! It involves a lot of patience and waiting (the actual birth itself, I mean). It is a natural process that usually will complete successfully in its own good time. 'Guy energy' – i.e. the normal and natural desire of men to 'do something' – to be active rather than receptive – to take control - is really at odds with this 'waiting game'. Modern medicine is very much in this masculine, controlling realm, and is just not the compatible kind of energy for birth. Of course, I acknowledge the occasional need for quick intervention. What I'm saying is that the male-oriented attitude makes this more likely, sooner, and in more cases. And once intervention happens, the mother, sadly, loses control.

I was very lucky to have about six women friends present at the birth and supporting me at various times. Four loving friends surrounded me when Cahya finally came (on the video you can see us chatting and joking between contractions). This support was invaluable and so empowering.

It surprises me that I have never found any description of what birth is actually like. Nowhere! And nobody explains what it means from a metaphysical viewpoint, so I shall try to do that here.

Everyone goes on about 'pain control' and obsesses over what drugs to use, but sorry, they are missing the point! The most important thing in my view is not 'pain control' but 'fear control'. Giving birth feels very like being on an ocean or in a big sea. Every so often, a big wave of sensation rolls over you. Just like swimming, it doesn't hurt being in the water, as long as you remember to breathe, relax, and don't tense up and get scared. Roll with the waves – don't panic, or you could go under and drown, just as in a real sea! The actual feeling is a bit like orgasm with a kind of wiggly tickly electric charge thrown in. Sorry that's the best I can do to describe it! But it didn't hurt.

Debra, our midwife, kept up a wonderful tirade of 'saying nice things' like 'the baby doesn't want to hurt you', 'it's safe to give birth' and 'it doesn't have to be for you like it was for your mother' and things like that. This made a vast difference to me. When Debra wandered off for a moment to supervise the birth pool, and I was left alone without this support, I found myself gazing into a vast dark abyss of fear – and I knew very well that that was where the pain was too. So I quickly called her back 'Debra! Come back and say 'nice things!' So she did and I was fine. I have great resources, a lot of yoga training which helps enormously with breathing and staying centred. Yet I could see clearly how I could have very easily lost it, stopped flowing with the process and started resisting and therefore feeling fear and hence pain. You MUST say 'yes' to the process.

Putu started getting sick at exactly the time Cahya was being born. We didn't know it, but he was coming down with chickenpox. Fortuitously, as the baby was taking a long time to come (the labour stalled at one point and was revived by using a drip – I'm not averse to modern things – I just want input and choice about when they are used!) Putu went off to his village in Tabanan to pray. Cahya was born at the moment of prayer, and luckily, this distance also kept her safe from the chickenpox.

Birth is a truly 'cosmic' experience. It is an intense moment of coming together of karma for both mother and baby. I believe the way in which the birth happens is largely down to the karma of the baby. The soul of the baby chooses how and when to come. Birth is probably the most vulnerable and lonely time of a woman's life (however good the support she has). The North American Indians believe that a woman journeys alone to the land of souls to pick up the soul of her baby and bring it back, and it certainly felt like that to me. A different state of consciousness is entered. A song I wrote, 'The Journey' aims to capture that feeling, and is reproduced here.

The Journey

I travelled to the land of snows
How you get there no-one knows
It's cold and white and no grass grows
I brought you back with me.

It's long and lonely in my coat
Reindeer fur and boots of goat
But I crossed over and this I wrote
I brought you back with me

I arrived tired and you were lying there
Naked on a bed of fur
I picked you up and held you here
I brought you back with me

I called your name and you awoke
Piercing eyes like steely smoke
You cried to me and something broke
I brought you back with me

It's a lonely journey in the night
But somehow all is filled with light
You're my tiny fire bright
You light my home for me.

Wave by wave
And breath by breath
Brings me to the land of death
To find your soul
and bring it back
Bring it back with me

Jeli Lala © 2000

I was able to 'channel' information from Cahya before she was born. It was great to have this connection! I asked her to make the birth easy and she said 'she'd do her best as far as she could'. During the birth, she told me she'd come at twelve o'clock. I thought this was to be in a couple of hours time (it was ten o'clock at night) but it turned out to be fourteen hours later (she was born at 11:59!) People also talk about birth in terms of 'how many hours' it lasts (the implication being that it's awful if it's long – I suppose because everyone believes it's painful). It was fine for me that Cahya took quite a long time – only a day to get a new life into the world doesn't seem so long to me!

The baby also told me of her previous life, as a male teacher of calligraphy on the border of China and Tibet. She certainly has a great affinity with drawing, and has always made calligraphic writing type squiggles from the moment she first picked up a pen! If you are pregnant, and want to try connecting with your baby, sit with pen and paper, relax and ask a question inwardly of the baby (it's fun to let your partner ask the questions) and just write down the first answer than comes.

After the birth, we were all completely exhausted. I have a photo of Putu stretched out, stiff as a board, clutching a broom from sweeping the floor, just zonked. He's smothered in white 'boré' – rice ground with deliciously fragrant flowers and mixed with water and put on the skin (a local remedy for the horrendous chickenpox blisters). He looks like a skinny deranged aborigine ghost! I wasn't much better – so tired – I hadn't realised what a massive physical impact birth has. In the days after the birth, the body releases litres and litres of excess water through the urine and does a huge adjustment process. There is a need to rest and on top of this, the new baby is in the bed and needs feeding, changing and constant attention! Giving birth is easy compared to the energy and time needed for caring for a child.

The three weeks after the birth, though, were a lyrical time turnaround between sleeping, washing nappies, listening to Robbie Williams, feeding, eating, sleeping, just watching the tropical garden outside, washing nappies... Getting to know each other and hanging out together were really nice luxuries.

And really, this has continued up to now. Having a child is a constant and never ending wheel of things that must be done (and done NOW!)

You may have heard the quote 'children give you patience'. I would like to change it to read 'children give you patience...because they can be the most incredibly annoying beings on the planet!' They quite naturally have no respect for your time boundaries, priorities or ideas! They need you and they always need you NOW!!! (At times I find myself just wishing I could go to the bathroom in peace without hearing 'MummmmEEEEEE!' coming at me through the door!) Though, as any parent will tell you, I wouldn't change it for the world. Nothing can compare with the joy of your child bringing you a flower for the first time, or saying 'thank-you' or giving you a great beaming smile or a hug. I've had to learn to let go of my priorities and try to focus on hers. (With varying success – the other 'given' quality of the parent seems to be that of guilt!).

The main thing I want for our child is to give her a strong sense of self-esteem. So, we don't make her 'wrong' if she makes a mistake. We don't yell at her, criticise her or hit her (this was normal practise in Western upbringing when I was a child). We certainly don't give her negative inputs like 'you're stupid!' etc. We often praise and encourage her. And we listen to what she wants (however idiosyncratic!) and allow it if possible.

Boundaries are challenging though – how do you control a screaming two year-old – set the boundary, not give in, yet try to minimise the size of the ensuing drama? I find this very difficult. The only answer I have so far is 'distraction!' Give the message, and then change the subject so it doesn't become too big a thing. I'm still working on this one! The relationship with one's child seems to magnify anything that is already difficult (giving great opportunity for practice!) The other 'given' of being a parent, of course, is knowing that you can only do your best, and you are bound to do some things wrong.

Perhaps the biggest thing I've learned from joining the parent clan is just how difficult it is even to provide the basic things like a nice place to live, clean clothes, good food on the table, time and attention – just this takes a huge amount of energy, never mind anything 'intangible' like love, support, a sense of self-worth... I now have much greater appreciation and gratitude for my own parents – they did their best in difficult circumstances. I have really let go of blaming them for anything disagreeable that happened when I was a child, and this feels like a great freedom.

If you are already a parent, salute! If you are planning to become one, congratulations – it's one of the greatest journeys there is. And if you're not in this realm, I hope you'll enjoy opportunities that come your way to spend time with children.

The Birth of my Son Riho by Anni Võhma from Estonia

I was 18 when I became pregnant for the first time. It was my first university year. I had been together with my partner for a couple of years. We loved each other deeply and after the first shock had passed, we were truly happy and excited about having a baby. Truth be told, I was even a bit relieved, because I had been studying really hard for the last four years and needed a break.

My mother and grandmother gave me a hard time, but I had some great friends and a wonderful man (with a big friendly family) by my side who gave me the support I needed. As I was at that age, where studying and looking for new information was very natural, I started learning everything I could about pregnancy and childbirth.

At first, I was terrified because of the pain I expected to experience during natural childbirth. You can't have an elective C-section in Estonia, so I started looking for the support I needed to give birth naturally and without fear. I wanted to enjoy the whole experience.

I knew I wanted to give birth in water. I was about 10 years-old when I read about the very first water births in Estonia and this seemed the gentlest way to greet your newborn child. I was still nervous about the pain. (*It is not fair to young women to be raised in a society where childbirth is firsthand associated with pain. I knew that this couldn't be all there was, there had to be a better way. I looked and found the support I needed, but what about all the women who don't?*)

I found a doula that had experienced an ecstatic childbirth and we met over a cup of tea. I was prepared to talk with more than one doula to find the one that fitted me best, but after ten minutes with Inge I was convinced I had already found the right one. She was also a SOURCE Breathwork therapist and we started meeting on a regular basis. Sometimes Ivar, my partner, joined us. He also liked her.

It was Sunday night and I had an appointment with my doctor the next day. I was almost two weeks over my due date. We had agreed that there was no need to speed up the process but, according to the hospital rules, she still had to check me to see if everything was alright.

It was about 9pm when I felt the first contractions. Ivar was asleep and I had just finished crying and sobbing "why won't he come out already"? The contractions were light and as I had already gone through one false alarm with light contractions, I didn't give it further thought. Ivar woke up. We cuddled a bit and at one point I noticed a tiny amount of blood. We both felt relieved and very excited, but neither of us thought I was in labour. We were hungry, so we went and bought all kinds of good stuff. When we were standing in the line I felt for the first time that things just might get serious, so I grabbed the last watermelon there was and a chocolate (I knew I wanted to have these foods when I gave birth, because one needs fluids and energy). Contractions became a bit stronger. I automatically started to breathe slower and deeper. Driving back from the store I decided to time the contractions – they were very regular 2 minutes apart. It was confusing, because I was told to go to the hospital when the rushes were 5 minutes apart, but it also let us know for sure, that this was it. I thought how cool it was that tomorrow at the same time there would already be three of us. Ivar was really happy too, because he was tired of waiting.

I told him to make a big bottle of wild thyme tea. (It helps to relax cervical muscles; I had picked it myself from the woods a couple of months earlier. I had also picked achillea from the meadows to help the uterus to contract after childbirth, but be careful - in big amounts it is known to make breast milk taste bitter.) I tried to eat so I would have enough energy in case it was a long birth (and it was), but the rushes got more intense and I had to focus all my attention to integrate them so instead of eating I ended up speed walking around the pool table, squeezing its every hole as I passed. I would have wanted to take this table with me to the hospital. I later found out that Ivar had cooked quite a meal for himself – luckily, because there was a long night ahead. When another rush started, I had to start speed walking again, because it would hurt if I stood still. When moving around I felt like a powerful ancient woman. In between rushes I talked very much and very fast. I think this was my way to cope with all this energy, I didn't know how to use it another way. I started using vocals to relax during the rushes. Haaaa... Huuuu... That's when Ivar called Inge, our doula, to come over. She came fast, all glowing and smiling. We went to our room on the third floor with her and gathered my things. I remember calculating the time very accurately so I would get downstairs between two rushes.

We had two huge bags full of our things – my own pillow, the watermelon, clothes for us and the baby, my laptop and the speakers to listen to music during birthing, lots of candles, a big bottle of herbal tea, a small plastic bathtub for the baby (in case I couldn't give birth in water I wanted to give him a bath afterwards to help him relax).

The welcome ceremony in hospital included a bit of an arrogant midwife and a CTG (the most annoying procedure during the whole thing). Dilation was four fingers wide. Then for some reason I had to stay in the corridor for quite a while, which was okay, because it was beautiful with lots of space to walk, make noises and be inspired by the wild screams of a Russian woman who was giving birth in one of the rooms. Ivar confessed later, that he was a bit worried about how that would affect me.

Months later I found out why we had to wait in the hall. They didn't want to give us their last free birthing room with a bathtub, because it was getting cleaned, but Inge overheard this and knowing how much I wanted to give birth in water she convinced them that we could wait. (That's why a woman shouldn't go to a hospital alone.)

So we went to birthing room no 4. It was 2am. There was a huge, deep, white heart-shaped bathtub. Ivar and Inge turned off the lights, lit the candles and put on some shaman drum music. I went to take a hot shower, also in candlelight. It felt good, cosy and beautiful. The rushes were getting stronger of course, but I was still enjoying all this. As running water was a wonderful relaxer, I stayed under the shower until my feet got tired, then they brought me a big rubber ball to sit on and I stayed for some time more. Occasionally Ivar or Inge looked into the bathroom, smiled and went away. Luckily, I got another midwife, a joyful woman with a wonderful strong Russian accent. She came to the room pleasantly rarely and as she saw that I was okay and very well taken care of, she never stayed for too long. She told me something supportive every time she was in the room, commented that I had a great ability to relax or that I had nice wide hips.

Inge prepared the bath and sinking my body into warm water felt like the ultimate pleasure, considering the situation. Rushes kept on coming about two minutes apart, it was a true marathon. As it was still night time and dark, I could enjoy it. It was dark, there were some candles, music, an ancient rhythm, for a while these together made a very sensual experience. A person was being born and I had two wonderful folks there supporting me in every way possible. It seemed as if at least one of them always knew intuitively what I needed and when their intuition wasn't quick enough I gave strict orders from my bathtub-throne like a queen frog: "Drink! Watermelon! Chocolate!"

Inge was telling me affirmations now and then like: "Your body is safe." or "We are doing this together." She assured me that my body and the baby's body are perfectly designed for this. Ivar was telling me how much he loves me and that I was doing great.

We created our own space there, and all the medical help was around the corner if I should need it. Now I know that although a mother can often CHOOSE a place to give birth, she can also take what's given and MAKE it her own, CREATE the perfect atmosphere. It happens almost by itself if the surrounding people are supportive, conscious and present.

I didn't even notice every time the midwife came in. I also didn't notice that I was often breathing very deeply and slowly, like during a breathing session, but I was later told I did. One time the midwife stepped in and as I was breathing and in my own bubble, she asked Inge: "She is breathing?" "Breathing." "Very nicely breathing," commented the midwife.

It was around 5 or 6 in the morning when it started to get lighter (the windows were huge and the curtains didn't cover much) and I was getting tired. I didn't like the light. I had hoped the child would be born before the sun came up, but it seemed that was not going to happen. At first, I felt a bit frustrated, but luckily the rushes got so heavy that I didn't even care about the light anymore. From about 6 to 7 I felt like giving up. 'I can't', 'I don't want to', 'I'm not able to'. 'I don't have any more strength'. 'Just take the baby out and let's call it a day'. It wasn't the pain that was hard to bare. The biggest challenge was feeling tired. Exhausted. A rush isn't just pain. That was surprising to me. Yes, there can be pain, but there is SO MUCH MORE. It is ENERGY, energy so enormous and mind blowing happening inside you. It is a variety of sensations – a hot flush, a contraction, a push, stretching, a rush of hormones that is constantly changing the way you feel, your level of consciousness. And this is very intense. When a rush is over, it is really completely over and you can feel fine, but the fear of "another one coming right up" didn't let me relax and rest.

As for me, it had been very intense for a long time now and, as I thought that birthing shouldn't be that hard, I asked for an epidural. Ivar's face changed immediately like I had done something wrong or something bad had happened. The midwife didn't think I needed one. She didn't want to refuse directly, so she tried to win time by saying that there was no anaesthetist available right now, but she'd let me know as soon as there was. Then, about 7 am she came to check me and told me that the dilation was so big (7-8 cm) that there was no point of giving me an epidural anymore. My mind was glad because I was well aware of the benefits of a natural childbirth and the side-effects of an epidural, but my body was very disappointed and wanted to cry. I think she probably lied a bit about the dilation, but I am very grateful to her about that little white lie. I did have the strength to bring my baby into this world naturally; somebody just had to press the right button.

I did feel small, helpless and sad for a while, but this passed, thanks to the active support from Inge and Ivar. If this is the way it's going to be, let it be. Rush after rush.

I was in the bathtub much longer than recommended by the doctors. I had to come out from time to time. The rushes became heavier right away, the pain became sharper, I felt naked and unprotected – well, I was naked. Going back to the water every time was such bliss.

Midwives shifted. We were lucky again. The second midwife was also great, joyful and supportive, although a bit too chatty. I was not in that state of mind where I wanted to think, talk or listen to questions. Ivar told me later that I looked exhausted, like a spawned herring.

It became so intense I could hardly bear it. And then even more intense. It was like this for an hour. There was a handrail above the bath, so when I was on my knees, I could put my hands up and hang there, swinging my body back and forth. Moving water massaged me with just the right pressure. Hot shower on my lower back, pressing the right spots on my wrists to relieve pain, staring into another person's eyes and roaring like a bear were surprisingly effective, especially the bear voices — they were nothing like screams of pain, but more like ancient animal sounds a woman is able to make only during childbirth to relax herself.

I felt I had taken with me exactly the right people. Inge was radiating one kind of energy and Ivar another kind, and together it was the perfect support. Not once did I have to explain, prove or beg. I was wholly accepted, acknowledged and honoured in my efforts.

It was about 9 or 10 o'clock when a doctor came in for the first time. He was by coincidence the father of my classmate. I knew that doctors only came when everything wasn't going as it should — in my case they were worried about the length of my labour. He checked me and asked me if he could break the water bag to speed up the process. I was lying on my back in the bed and didn't feel like a woman giving birth, but more like a patient who should probably agree with her doctor - so I agreed. The waters were a bit greenish. The hospital rules said that when the waters are green, a woman is not to give birth in the water, so my midwife attempted to keep me on dry land for "just a little bit longer", but she obviously didn't try hard enough, because I was back in my bathtub in no time. The doctor had left. The rushes started turning into pushes. The midwife gave me an Oxytocin pill to put under my tongue, so the uterus wouldn't get tired just before the finish. That's what they have to do after opening the water bag. She also did a CTG. Although I was standing up during the CTG, it still felt like torture, because I couldn't move myself the way I wanted to.

When the rushes turned into pushes, it got a lot easier, but the sensation of something huge moving down inside me was very scary at first. I needed to tell myself repeatedly that my body was safe, because the way my body was making room for the baby to come out felt so powerful. Rushes somewhat resemble menstrual cramps, but I had experienced nothing that felt like the pushes. I was afraid that my baby was too big for my hips, but soon I felt that he was moving down, so there had to be enough space and I wasn't scared anymore.

I wanted to touch his head, but instead I felt something weird and wrinkly. The midwife checked and told that it's okay, this is the head, but there is not very much space, the head is being moulded right now and the skin is wrinkly. This was the first time I touched my baby.

The midwife started "leading the birth", told me what to do, how to breathe (I listened to that part), when to press (I ignored what she said about pressing and let my body decide). I was in a totally different level of consciousness, like I was an animal in a human's world, unable to communicate in words. It was very instinctive, like a part of my brain had turned off and another one was working double. I think I said something, but I didn't understand my own words. Losing control about how socially acceptable my behaviour was or wasn't, I bit Inge's hand. That very moment I "came back" for a second, realized that I had another person's hand in my mouth, so I quickly opened my jaws and pulled away. I actually wanted to bite my own hand, but it was busy holding on to the edge of the bathtub. I felt the more upright the position I took, the easier it felt. If the bathtub had been deeper I would have done it standing up, but I did it on my knees instead.

The moment the head crowned, I made a high pitched scream. Then I asked if the baby was out now. He wasn't. The midwife was applying slight pressure to the baby's head, he was a big baby and she wanted to give me time to stretch. With the next push he came all out – the head and the body at the same time. I couldn't tell when the head came out, but I felt when the little body was sliding through me and this felt almost pleasurable compared to what I had felt a minute ago.

The baby and the midwife were behind me, so I didn't see them right away, but I heard Ivar being thrilled and repeating: "He is here. He is here. He is here." When I turned around I first noticed Ivar's face and his expression was something I can't describe. Everything was so magical. It felt like time was enormously speeding up, every second was so valuable and over so soon. Now he was 10 seconds old... 11, 12, 13, 14...

He was so beautiful and small and purple and slippery and I didn't even know how to hold him, because he was so beautiful and small and slippery. They gave us a soft warm towel to cover him up and we stayed in the bathtub skin-to-skin for a while. He made a couple of loud cries to clean the lungs but there was no desperate crying. I was amazed by the cord – it was a beautiful bright shade of light blue. When it stopped pulsating, Ivar cut it.

Ivar took his shirt off and held the child skin-to-skin on his chest until I came out from the bathtub. I was cold and went straight to the bed, under a warm blanket. Of course I took Riho with me and he started nursing. He was so beautiful. I had seen many newborns in videos and I knew that a baby who has just come through a birth canal can look rather weird, but he really was beautiful.

The placenta was born and they asked if we would like to take it with us. I said no, and please don't even show that thing to me, but the next second I changed my mind and said okay, bring it here, I want to see it. It looked weird to me. They gave me a couple of stitches. At first I was scared of the placenta, but actually it was easy.

They then gave us time to be with each other. I completely lost track of time. At some point Riho was weighed and measured. When he was put on the baby-scale, he looked at his father and SMILED for the very first time. Of course he had a good reason for that - he weighed 10 pounds!

The most important thing I learned is that, if possible, DO NOT make decisions when lying on your back in a hospital bed. A mother shouldn't receive any questions in that position, because this is the position of a patient, of an ill person, and if there is a doctor in the room, a woman can easily feel that there is something wrong with her and agree with unnecessary intervention. If a decision has to be made, take your time, stand up or at least stay on all-fours and feel your own strength. If everything is alright, you have time. You don't have to push if your body doesn't feel like pushing. Your body will do it by itself when the time is right.

When it gets really intense, it is easy to forget that there is another conscious human being involved – the baby. She is also hearing and feeling everything and deserves your support and attention. It is good if somebody reminds you from time to time, that you are doing this together. Talking to the baby can be a tremendous source of strength for both of you. Your baby deserves to be welcomed gently and worthily.

Birth of Daughter Kertu by Anni Võhma

Second Birth

I planned to give birth in Tartu, in the same amazing obstetrical department where my son was born, 115 miles away from home. It was about 2-3 hour drive. We were aware I might have to give birth in the car. For many reasons it still seemed to be a better place than our local hospital.

Two days before the delivery I visited my midwife and she guessed I was about to give birth very soon. She told me that she hadn't seen a baby "so low and ready to go", for a long time.

Tuesday evening I got bored and carefully repacked the hospital bag. The next morning about 5am I woke up after a good night's sleep and realized that the water sack had broken. Half an hour later it became clear that rushes had also started; they came two minutes apart and became more intense really fast. I called doula Inge and my personal midwife Margit, so they would go to the obstetrical department (they both lived much closer) and make everything ready for our arrival. We also called the grandparents-to-be. About an hour later, we took off with a grandiose plan to make a stop where my parents-in-law lived to pick up a babysitter for our year-and-a-half-old son Riho, make me a bottle of wild thyme tea (to relax the cervical muscles), switch our car to a bigger one and get to Tartu before the baby was born.

When we got to my parents-in-law, I started using vocals "aa" and "uu" to help me relax. I didn't go into the house; instead I started speed-walking around the car. While Ivar was dealing with exchanging cars and making thyme tea, I was accompanied by a big wolf dog. It must have been quite a sight as we were howling together in the dark. It was January with lots of snow everywhere.

Soon all four of us got into the car; I was kneeling in the front seat, howling louder and louder, as the journey went on. Riho didn't seem to understand what was happening. I told him that mommy was singing his sister out. He compassionately imitated my "aa's" and "uu's" for a while and then decided he'd better sleep at this confusing time. The babysitter, Ivar's younger sister, was dealing with the phone and the tea-bottle. Ivar was focused on driving fast and properly. At that time I felt most supported by the thought "we are doing this together", so I quietly repeated it to myself and gave baby my attention.

The rushes got really intense really fast, so after 30 miles I felt for the first time that we were probably not going to get to the hospital, yet we continued driving. I wanted really badly to get into the tub or at least take a shower – a wish that didn't go away during the labour. I called Inge, breathed with her, made some loud bear sounds during rushes and muttered about epidural in between. Although the pose I was in was very good, it was so hard not being able to move around. I fractiously planned never again to give birth, talk about birth, commune with breathers, doulas or midwives, and to give away all my books related to the topic. (And now I'm studying to become a midwife myself...)

Inge told me that it was probably late for an epidural now - which was true as I was probably in transition phase - and she brought me back to positive thinking which was definitely the most supportive thing to do. So I started saying "Jaaaaaaa!" ("Yes!" in Estonian) during rushes. I realized that in one way or another, I was probably going to give birth in the car. I wasn't fond of the idea, but I felt really supported - someone was there for me, fully present, focused on this birth. Also, someone was taking care of the rest of the important stuff - Riho and driving.

Suddenly I shouted: "Inge, I need to push!" (We were still connected on the phone). Now it became obvious, that we wouldn't make it to Tartu; on the other hand, I knew that the transition phase – the hardest, most painful part for me - was soon going to end. The phone was given from one to another. Ivar remained totally calm. As we had to choose between two hospitals, one of which was in Tartu, he decided to aim for that one and call the ambulance to meet us half way. Our midwife had also already notified the ambulance, that there was a woman in labour moving towards Tartu – and really fast.

I twisted myself into a position, where my shoulders could be lower than my hips, to slow the labour down a bit. I could feel the baby's head in my birth canal with my fingers, so I placed a clean pillow under me and took off my boots and jeans, so the baby wouldn't get stuck in them. I also asked her to wait a bit. It's good we didn't spot any police patrols – a car speeding at 80 miles per hour with a naked butt in the front seat would have surely caught their attention.

Meanwhile we received blessings from our friends Binnie, Lembe and Iida-Leena via phone. It was so supportive to hear that they were thinking of us and meditating.

We met the ambulance at about 8 o'clock. They didn't seem to be very clever, as they were asking every question at least twice and making every suggestion thrice. Now I had to start fighting for my every wish. When I got out of the car, they didn't allow me to walk to the ambulance car myself (ten steps at the most), instead I had to get on their trolley so they could roll me in. I didn't have my boots on, just socks, and standing on an icy road I didn't argue, got onto the trolley and kneeled there, waiting. This was also not to their liking, as they wanted me to lie down on that thing, barely two feet wide. I got angry and sent them where the sun doesn't shine. So they had to roll me in this way. Ivar also came in for a couple of minutes, but as there was not much space and the paramedics still hoped to make it to Tartu, we started driving again. At first, Ivar tried to follow us but the ambulance drove off at about 95 miles per hour.

The paramedics repeatedly tried to convince me that if I lay down, it would be easier for them to help me. I answered with bear sounds, and if that didn't seem to get my point across, I told them that this was my second delivery and I knew being in that position was easier for me. This didn't convince them either, but they didn't force me this time. After I got to the ambulance, the most intense part, where rushes and pushes came simultaneously, still lasted for a while – and, of course, this was the time those clever women picked to ask me about my personal data, address and so on. Oh well, their argument "but we have to fill in the forms!" was basically stronger than my "right now I'm not talking to youuuuuuuuuuuuuuuuuu!" They got their damn data.

I tried on the oxygen mask and it was really helpful at first, but it soon started to bother me and I took it off. Next thing they didn't like were my bear sounds. I was told that I should breathe out quickly and quietly. As my deep breathing and noises felt very right and supportive to me, I told them I was better this way and continued to do my thing. But they thought I simply hadn't understood them and explained to me the same thing over and over again until I sent them to where the sun don't shine - again. I didn't mean to be rude, I just wanted them to stop talking and that was the only thing that seemed to shut them up.

As they thought we had plenty of time, we stopped at a local first-aid station, where a petite blond woman finished her night shift and a big brunette one joined us.

As I was fighting against all their suggestions, they finally gave up, sat down with baffled faces, hands on their laps, and asked, how they could help me. (That's the spirit!) I told them to turn off the lights, speak quietly and use the term "rush", not a "birthing pain". I got what I had asked for, and further communication became much easier and friendlier.

Rushes had stopped and pushes, although overwhelming and immensely powerful, were to my surprise, absolutely painless. There were sensations of warmth, pressure and stretching, massive rushes of energy but no pain whatsoever. I was kneeling on this jolly orange trolley and felt stupendously empowered. I held on to whatever handles I could reach (there was a lot of them and probably not all were meant for holding on to) and breathed deeply. During pushes I was rocking myself slightly back and forth. The walls of the car were covered with wires and machinery. The car was jolting a lot, although the women repeatedly told the driver to be more careful. The jolting didn't bother me at all; actually, this powerful vibration was quite relaxing.

The next thing we disagreed on was whether I should be in my current position or lie down. They told me to "rest and save my strength". I told them I had had a good night's sleep, my current position was perfect and the baby was coming out right away – exactly for what should I save my strength? They seemed impervious to my words and kept repeating to me to lie down and rest. They even wanted to put a pillow under my head. The pillow of course soon found itself on the floor. Maybe they were just afraid I would fall off the narrow trolley?

At one point I felt my tissues stretching strongly and burning a little, so I shouted to the woman who had to catch the baby: "She's coming!", and as I had said it, the baby forcefully moved downwards. I heard them being truly surprised: "Oh, she is showing herself already!" - And the baby moved back up again. They really hadn't paid attention to what I was saying about the pushes and baby being born soon, and hadn't thought the delivery was so far along. Our driver was told to quickly turn off the highway and stop the car. The first turn-off leads us to Mustvee's old military airfield in the middle of nowhere. We parked just at the beginning of the runway, and that's the place Kertu was born. As she was being born I could tell that this one would be much smaller than my first baby. The head came out with a couple of pushes and then I felt like I was giving birth in some typical movie where they shout: "Now push! Push!! Push!!!" Why should I push when I didn't feel like pushing at that moment? The delivery was happening so quickly, that I had no intention of pushing until I tore apart, so I didn't push along at all and breathed through all the pushes. I don't know if they pulled a little or whether the baby wriggled herself, but then I felt weird wriggling sensations inside the birth canal and out she was. It was 8:25am. To calm the nerves of the paramedics, she made some energetic noises that soon turned into the babbling characteristic of a newborn. I told them to lower their voices and give the baby to me without cutting the cord. I had to repeat it a couple of times. As there was little space to move myself, she was passed to me through my legs. I quickly took off the rest of my clothes, bowed over her and held her as tightly against my body as I could in that peculiar position. She tried to look around, but the lights were switched on again and too bright, so I told the paramedics to turn them off – that's when they thought I was ashamed to be naked in front of strangers.

She opened her eyes and looked at me. I found myself drowning into her eyes and silently explaining to her the most important things in the world about love, while giving the paramedics a short, but at that moment necessary lecture on how the newborn's ears and eyes were not used to such strong stimulation, and there was no need to scare her. Then we were given some precious peaceful moments, but not too many, as we disagreed whether or not they should cut the cord. It was still pulsating strongly. Our argument was like this: "Let's cut the cord now", "No, it is still pulsating". "How about now?" "No". "Now?" "No". "Now?" "No" (and so on...)!

The male driver stood up for me by saying to them magisterially that there was plenty of time and we could wait. I briefly explained to them, why it was so important not to cut the cord too early. They really listened and asked me if I was a medic, too. I smiled. Finally the contractions started again, and as Kertu seemed to be breathing nicely on her own, I let them cut the cord. Before they did, they looked outside of the window to see if the father was already there. He wasn't. So we lay down on the trolley, cuddling, Kertu started on her very first breakfast and we started driving again. The placenta was born somewhere on the road.

When everything calmed down, the women admitted that they had been quite nervous, as they had only attended three births and if something had gone wrong, they had no special equipment in the car to help the baby. In bigger towns there is usually an ambulance car that is meant for taking care of newborns.

In the meantime, everything and everybody was good and ready in Tartu. Midwife and doula were waiting, a delivery room with a bathtub was ready, Ivar was driving around the parking lot, trying to find a place to park. The only thing missing was the woman in labour. Everybody was really confused for some time. They had no idea where I was, in what condition and what was taking us so long because I had left my cell phone in our car. Finally, my trolley was rolled into the department where my whole team greeted me joyfully at the door. I felt so very welcome, and everybody was so amused and happy. The paramedics had tremendously proud faces on them, like they had been the ones giving birth. There was a little fuss in the room as the ambulance wanted their sheets back, but these were wrapped around me and the baby was nursing and I didn't want to interrupt her. After a while we moved from the trolley to a bed, the paramedics got their sheets and left. I must have looked rather comical as I had nothing on but streaked knee-high socks with separate toes.

Our midwife gave us all the time we needed and told me that she was not even going to measure the baby as the doctor would do it anyway afterwards. I am deeply grateful to her for everything. She only checked the baby's breathing and if I needed any stitches – I didn't. Right after that Riho, Ivar and our babysitter arrived. Riho was very curious about his little sister, but also tired, and soon they took him to sleep. We stayed with Inge. I took a nice hot shower that I had longed for since the very beginning and she looked after the baby. As I left her sight, the baby started crying a bit, but Inge told her, that mother was just around the corner and would be back soon – and just as she said that, she stopped crying, took a deep breath and calmed down.

Before we got to our family-room, the doctor had to check and measure the baby. 50 cm, 3770 grams, everything worked properly. They were astonished how vivacious I was; one doctor even asked me if I was really the mother. I was very surprised, too – I could walk and sit almost like there hadn't been a birth, the belly had pulled back a lot and I was overflowing with energy and joy and pride and gratitude.

Looking back I feel blessed I could give birth without CTGs and vaginal exams. I understand that they give vital information about the baby's condition and the progress of childbirth. Nevertheless, they are terribly difficult to bear during strong rushes. I was confident because the baby was moving herself a lot throughout the birth, and the progress was just obvious. Although I couldn't move around at all and my legs became really stiff in the end, I was in the best possible position for me all the time and didn't have to lie down on my back, not even for a moment. I felt I was totally in charge of what was happening, although I couldn't fully focus on this birth as I had to fight for all my wishes. On the other hand, all this fuss and fighting made me feel like some kind of an almighty primordial woman and I was able to give birth calmly even when nothing went as planned, my helpers were nervous themselves, and there was no familiar or pleasant person next to me. It was not about what came from outside, but how I managed to support myself on the inside.

For me it was a truly powerful co-creation with my daughter. And when we arrived at the hospital, I was given so much care and love from the people who I wanted to be present at the birth; it didn't feel like I had missed out on anything. This experience was priceless for me. Now I know how empowering giving birth can be!

Some thoughts by Anni Võhma

Second Birth

Both days I gave birth are the most miraculous days of my life. It isn't always easy to take care of a newborn, but remembering the amazing experience we had gone through, helped me to keep it together. It was and is my 'happy place', eternal source of inner strength and empowerment.

And that is the way it should be – a birthing experience shouldn't be a factor that causes postpartum depression, it should keep the depression away.

I think her man and her doula make a great support for a woman in labour. A woman in labour shouldn't have to worry about organizing something or fighting for her rights. It is their duty - while one is taking care of the mother, the other one can take care of other things if necessary. Sometimes it can come to a situation where mother and newborn must be separated. It is good if one of them can go with the baby and another one can stay and take care of the mother.

A woman, who has given birth and enjoyed it, makes a great doula.

It can do a family good when a man sees his woman giving birth and his children being born and a woman can receive his loving support. I like how Cara, one of the Farm midwives in the book Spiritual Midwifery by Ina May Gaskin, said: "Over and over again, I've seen that the best way to get a baby out is by cuddling and smooching with your husband. That loving, sexy vibe is what puts the baby in there, and it's what gets it out, too".

It is funny how people think that giving birth has nothing to do with sexuality, although it involves the same hormones, similar brain activity and same body parts.

Pregnancy is a wonderful time to get to know yourself better. Things come up more easily; old memories, beliefs and secret potentials reveal themselves. It would be wise to use the opportunity.

A hospital CAN be a very good place to give birth. For me it is not about the place where the birth takes place, but about the people who are there.

Please, do not forget the baby! Be gentle and listen AND respond. Before birth, during birth, after birth. Usually there is no need to shock the baby with bright lights, loud high-pitch voices, cold air, absence of mother's smell and heartbeat, and ignoring his attempts to communicate and achieve skin-to-skin, eye-to-eye contact.

And do not forget the fathers. They can feel a bit left out during pregnancy when their lady seems to be the centre of the Universe. Actually it is new and interesting for them too, and they can be just as eager to learn new things and in need of some support. A man who has received enough support during his woman's pregnancy can make a wonderful supporter during childbirth.

Women should NOT feel bad about having an epidural, C-section or not enjoying the birth.

Zenya's birth by Lynne Thorsen

Author, Self-Healing Facilitator, Empowered Birth Educator
www.lynnethorsen.com

My pregnancy with my first child, in 2001, was one of the most wonderful times in my life. I had finished working a few weeks before getting pregnant and this allowed me a unique time of self-indulgence, being time rich and being able to focus my attention on the growing being inside me.

I exercised by running, playing tennis, playing golf and going to pre natal yoga. I improved my nutrition giving up tea and coffee and eating lots of oily fish, vegetables and fruit. I ignored the advice to avoid cheese, peanuts or cold meats. I drank alcohol minimally and only after thirteen weeks. In the latter stages, I drank raspberry leaf tea and did perineal massage to assist in not tearing.

I meditated and did visualisations to assist in both pregnancy and the birth preparation. During these sessions I would focus on connecting with the baby inside me.

Although unaware of my creativity during pregnancy, I see now that I was being very creative. I renovated and painted much of the inside of our house and I wrote a thesis for my holistic therapist qualification, which is a great piece of writing.

I was preparing for a homebirth with the local community midwives but during a home check up at thirty two weeks, my preparation received a setback when the midwife informed me that my baby was in the breech position and if she stayed that way, I would not be able to have a homebirth and a caesarean would be recommended.

Initially devastated by this news, I became convinced that she would turn and everything would be ok, however I started to research all I could about breech birth on the internet. At 35 weeks, she still had not turned, so I began interviewing independent midwives and I engaged the services of two wonderful midwives to assist my preparation. They suggested I go to an acupuncturist to assist in turning the baby. For four weeks my husband and I tried using mosh sticks (smells like marijuana) on the outside of my little toes to convince our baby to turn. I did shoulder stands and other physical positions to convince her to turn. Finally, the midwife said she could come with me to the acupuncturist and try to manually turn the baby whilst I was receiving the treatment. Twice she managed to get her bum up out of my pelvis and twice my baby sat straight back down again. The midwife declared, 'she does not want to turn, we are going to have a breech birth.'

She asked me to attend the local hospital and get a scan so that we could determine what position she was in and how big she was. Getting a scan required me to have an appointment with a hospital obstetrician. He lectured me on my choices to birth at home and ended with "Well if you want to risk the life of your unborn child..." My rage erupted and I stormed out of there furious at his ignorance and insensitivity.

In many ways the birth was textbook, going into labour on my due date and the contractions progressed exactly the way described by the birth professionals. After several hours of mild contractions, the intensity and length increased so that I no longer could sit down. I had to move around and sway my hips. Just as we went to bed, I lost the mucous plug and I knew that the birth was imminent. My husband was in denial as he did not like the idea of losing a night's sleep. I tried to go to sleep, but I had to get up every 10 minutes to move through the contractions. Shortly afterwards my waters broke and I told my husband to get out of bed and get the birthing pool ready. We called the midwife and my friend who had agreed to support at the birth. They both agreed to come over. By the time the midwife had arrived, I was 5 centimetres dilated and able to get into the birthing pool. The warm water felt wonderful, supporting my swollen belly through the contractions. Simultaneously, my husband read visualisations to me so that I could focus my attention away from the intensity of the contractions. Both worked brilliantly and labour continued to progress beautifully. In no time at all I was fully dilated and in transition.

At this stage the midwives asked me to get out of the birthing pool as they felt they could support the birth more effectively this way. It is the one thing that I would change about this birth as I believe the pool would have created more support for me during this life changing experience. My second stage continued for over two hours. The sheer power and energy of those 'pushing' contractions brought up fear in me. I thought that if I surrendered to their power, my body would tear in two. Eventually the fear of going to hospital outweighed the fear of splitting in two so I surrendered and that was when her bottom began to appear. A bottom is smaller than a head and in some ways this makes a breech birth easier as it is like a wedge, where the smaller part makes the way for the bigger part. Once her bottom was born each leg fell out and her body descended. The difference with a breech birth is that you have to birth the whole baby. Once her shoulders were out, her mouth appeared and she immediately breathed. The midwife said, "Fantastic we can all relax now!" That was ok for her to say, I still had a bowling ball to deliver. My perineum stretched beautifully and in no time I had birthed her head with no tears or stitches required.

The joy was immense for everyone involved and I was amazed at how the discomfort immediately disappeared. We embraced and welcomed our new little girl with an enormous sense of satisfaction and achievement. Ten minutes later, my stomach undulated like a wave and the placenta burst forth with the midwives only just managing to catch it in the bowl. Third stage also complete with no drugs or intervention.

What helped me to have this wonderful birth outcome was:

Knowledge
Belief in the female body to birth
Physical and mental preparation
Support from my husband, midwives, mother and friend
Methods to focus my attention away from pain
Great Focus and Intention

My top tip for a more pleasurable birth is focus your intention on joy and ecstasy and remove fear from your thought patterns.

Further Reading on Birth Stories

I would like to recommend the book *Spiritual Midwifery* by Ina May Gaskin because half the book is dedicated to positive birth stories, most of which the author actually attended personally as a midwife and birth supporter.

Poem For Jude

(For my son who was born on 15th January 2000 by Alexandra Florschutz, May 2000).

May my heart be forever open
And never disappointed.

May my ears always listen
Not to my own words.

May my eyes see beyond your disguises
Never accepting face value.

May I speak kind words of comfort
So you can sing again.

May my shoulder be there in times of need
To keep you strong.

May my hand lead you on life's bright path
And show you the cave of jewels.

May you then believe in life's rich treasures
As you my darling are my dear treasure.

May my feet stay firmly on the ground
But our spirits soar higher than rainbows.

May my opinions be un-judgemental
And rejoice in your every idea.

May my advice be unbiased and objective
And my hopes kept to myself.

May I always support your endeavours
As we journey through life together.

May I never hold you prisoner
But my trust set you free.

May you show me once more the magic of childhood
Now lost in the shadows of time.

May I show you happiness in sadness
May you believe in my everlasting love for you.

WOMAN

(By Alexandra Florschutz, 28th September 2011)

All women are varying designs of the same template.
All unique and perfect.

Some bear the souls of the future and others journey on a carefully pre assigned thoughtful path.
There is no right or wrong.

The tree that bears fruit after the blossom knows no other way but the tree that bears no fruit, may still have a fruitful life.

The moment a girl feels the gentle moist trickle of blood, sent to her from the moon, she knows her time has come.

She may now ascend into the realms of the sacred, sexual, potential mother – being a woman.

The moon hands her the key of life.
If it is her destiny to unlock the garden of maternal dreams she will find her way.

The paths that women tread are their own bitter sweet tales.

The pain at not conceiving after many moons of desire, is a slow burning torture that fills the soul with sorrow.
Or the loss of a life so treasured that no prayer or arm may comfort the years of empty gazes.

The day the moon turned her back, during the greatest hour, holds no light anymore.

When she beams down her silver rays, it is merely a silver disc, not a tide shifter or a moon cycle.

And there are women who have never felt the gentle caress of Love.
Nor the innocence of their own body or sexuality.
They yearn to know the path of the goddess.
The one who dances with light steps and a carefree will.

For some innocence is destroyed like an unforeseen cloud that spills a thousand rain drops of blood.
The blood that stains the wonders of the world, the internal dreams of women.

Thoughts that pounce like packs of wolves that rip the very hope from their heart.

Howling to the moon in jeers of rotten madness, as she stares, unblinking at the illusion of our suffering.

While others joyfully treasure the freedom of years.
Wisdom is their reward for the delicate growing, the passing of years, the work, the dedicated unconditional love.
For now they run free, naked in the meadow once more... not in naive carefree abandon but in sexual freedom.

Cured from the shame of self consciousness and once more reclaiming the golden horns of Isis.

Women of years rejoice in your freedom.
Stand tall, dance your merry dance, and let your wrinkles tell the world your story.
May you be honoured for blazing the trails for the ones that follow.

Women of all ages and all experience hold high the flag of the Feminine spirit.
Be the kiss that wakes you up from the eternal slumber.
Love the gift of inspiration that is our birthright.

Connect with our other half, our divine masculine.
Transform all thoughts into life-enhancing magic.
Love the divine beings that we are, each and every one of us.

We are leading the way for the children of tomorrow.
We carry the torch for the mothers of today.
We sing from the roof tops to the beauty of the mature.
We are taking life pleasurably into our own hands.
ALL Women, join hands and walk proudly next to the great Earth Mother who is our Heart.

Practical Tools for Birth

Thoughts to Remember

For an easier labour and birth by Binnie A. Dansby

Thoughts to Remember for an easier labour and birth by Binnie A. Dansby
www.binnieadansby.com

For pregnant women, their partners, and all who support birth with love.

- Be with people who think you can do it. Keep numbers to a minimum, and to people with whom you are familiar.

- Labour is active. Keep moving as long as you can. I don't mean you have to keep standing, just be as normal as possible, moving and being in positions that are comfortable. When you have a contraction, lean forward on someone or the wall or a chair. On your hands and knees is a good position to try, and I have noticed that the majority of the women who have given birth with me have done so on hands and knees.

- You know your body better than anyone, and if you 'listen in', you will know exactly what to do, even when you think you don't. Ask your partner or support person to remind you and to see to it that you are asked before anyone makes a decision about what you 'should' do. SLOW DOWN, take your time. You can also take the time to 'listen in' to your baby.

- Don't try to be strong, talk about how you are feeling and what you are thinking. When you can access your feelings, whatever they are, you can then use the energy however you choose. Make the sounds that are comfortable for you. You and your baby are the ones who matter, the ones everyone is there to support!

- Breathing is very helpful, and holding your breath is not. You will know how to breathe, for you. Keep relaxing your jaw, and opening your throat and pay attention to the breath. 'As above, so below'. The mouth and jaw and throat represent the pelvis and the birth canal. It is enough to do to pay attention 'above'; 'below' is perfectly designed to birth a baby.

- You always have a choice about what you Speak Out, no matter how your body is feeling. 'NO' causes the body to contract, and 'YES' causes the body to open. It may sound silly, and 'Yes' and 'Thank You' with a contraction will support you to stay focused on what is really important. I have seen it seem to work miracles.

- YOUR BABY IS FULLY CONSCIOUS AND EDUCABLE WHICH MEANS THAT SHE IS LISTENING AND COMMUNICATING TELEPATHICALLY. TALK TO HER; LET HER KNOW WHAT IS HAPPENING FOR YOU. UNDER ALL CIRCUMSTANCES, MAKE SURE THAT ANYTHING THAT IS DONE TO HER BE EXPLAINED TO HER FIRST.
IF YOU HAVEN'T ALREADY, TAKE SOME TIME EACH DAY TO LISTEN

TO YOUR BABY. REMEMBER THAT THIS BEING LOVES YOU BEYOND ANYTHING THAT YOU CAN EVEN IMAGINE! YOUR JOB IS TO OPEN TO RECEIVE ALL THE LOVE THAT SHE HAS FOR YOU AND YOUR PARTNER! THAT IS ALL YOUR BABY WANTS OR EVER WILL WANT.

- After the birth, see to it that you and your baby are together, or that she is with your partner. Make sure that you receive nurturing and support in physical forms. The baby and you are one unit; things don't change just because she is outside now. This doesn't mean that you can't put her down; just that you know that you need baby as much as baby needs you. You need to be cared for so that you can give what is needed.

- Choose an overall focus for yourself for the birth. Expansion is one that I know has been very successful. Another woman chose to think of her labour and birth as a sensual, sexual experience. Opening like a flower is wonderful. Pictures of full-blown roses and the lotus are images that are helpful. What images and aromas give you a sense of completion and wholeness and comfort?

- Allow yourself to receive all the love and support that is around you. Make clear choices and then trust that you make the right choices for you and your family. YOU DESERVE TO BE SURROUNDED BY PEOPLE WHO ARE LISTENING TO YOU AND THE BABY. PEOPLE WHO ARE SUPPORTING YOU TO HAVE AN EMPOWERED, ENLIGHTENING EXPERIENCE. THERE IS NO RIGHT OR WRONG WAY, IF YOU ARE LISTENING TO YOURSELF AND TO YOUR BODY. YOU HAVE EVERY THING THAT YOU NEED! HAVE AN INNOCENT, ECSTATIC TIME! I LOVE YOU.

Archetypal Affirmations For Conception, Pregnancy, Birth and Life

There is plenty of research into the power of our thoughts which seem to mirror a reality back to us. However, when thoughts combine with our energy, they magnify and we experience symptoms and behaviours in our physical reality as a consequence. Negative perceptions of ourselves and the world can be very debilitating if we don't try to untangle the origins of the thoughts that led us to make decisions about a situation in our past. If we work with Archetypal Affirmations, we may discover what is hidden in our unconscious and therefore change negative patterns into life-enhancing ones.

The colourful Archetypal Affirmations below, created by Binnie A Dansby, help to support our inner struggles with life, and are particularly helpful for pregnancy and birth. Dansby discovered that people seemed to have similar negative thought patterns, like recurring stories, that affected their lives and so, she created a positive alternative through affirmations that are linked to the Chakra system. Her CD, *Rhythm of Life*, contains the affirmations along with great music based on an ancient African mother rhythm.

"The affirmation will support all that is unlike itself to arise in order to be released. Affirmations are points of contemplation, thoughts you intend to bring into reality in your life. It is a thought form you intend to have become a real experience for you" (Dansby, B. A.)

- I am Earth

- I am Creativity

- Life only produces life

- The Breath is safe

- The Breath supports the release of discomfort, no matter how long I have held it

- My body is safe, no matter how I might be feeling

- The entire physical universe exists to support me in physical form

- I am surrounded by love and support from everyone in my life

- The more I let go and relax, the more I experience the support that is here for me

- All of my feelings are safe

- I am the power and the authority in my life

- I am the one who chooses what to think and how to use my Life Energy

- I am enough

- I do enough

- I have enough

- Everyone is glad that I am here

- Everyone is safe with me

- I am the innocent child of a Gentle Universe, I deserve to experience all of my love

- I am open to receive all the love and blessings that come to me

- I have a right to be here

- I am an expression of love

- It is safe to express myself fully and freely

- My expression is WELCOME

- My timing is perfect

- I am always in the right place at the right time, doing and saying the right thing

- I am connected in love to all that lives and all that breathes

- I am connected to Divine Intelligent that knows my good

- I am Spirit manifest in beautiful form

- I am a high thought, I am love

A Final Word

Our creativity is essential for maintaining a balanced existence and I certainly would not be without it. I have painted ever since my son was a baby, having a large exhibition when he was only nine months old. Painting keeps me alive, happy and sane as my life has not been straight forward at times. I have charted my creative journey over the years and noticed how it has reflected my personal development in a remarkable way. Having an outlet for unconscious thoughts and feelings is really helpful for all human beings whether pregnant or not although it can really help connect us with our impending birth. I would definitely explore my next pregnancy and any subsequent pregnancies despite my positive first experience because I know that other potential worries would have popped up in the meantime. I hope I have given you much food for thought and some helpful exercises to work through in your own time. It is paramount for women to take time out for themselves in order to stay connected to their pleasure. If you build a relationship with your pleasure, then it will see you through any situation. Art can help you as it is a pleasurable thing to do and as long as you don't judge yourself, especially for your technical skill, then it will be an enlightening experience. You can also do the exercises now even if your experience was many years ago – it is never too late.

Pregnancy and birth are deeply instinctual experience and part of nature spanning millions of years, an art with which we are rapidly losing touch. How do we reconnect back to the ancient natural life cycles of the human being and translate them, in a positive way, to our time? There needs to be adequate support for women to get back in touch with their intuitive side, like the archetypal creator woman, by exploring their non verbal and unconscious psyche. There are many different perspectives to each woman's life, her circumstances and her past, so one can never generalise or give a complete picture, but perhaps if we re-established a relationship with nature, the spiritual or mystical and not just the physical and medical side of pregnancy, then most births might not be so difficult for both mother and baby. I have made comparisons between art being the physical representation of our unconscious world and birth providing the bridge between the invisible to the visible. I believe that each individual can take active responsibility for transforming the current paradigm towards a more holistic approach to pregnancy and birth which will, over time, become a global change.

'Nothing ever goes away until it teaches us what we need to know' (Pema Chodron).

'You must be the change you wish to see in the world'! (Gandhi).

YES... YOU CAN DO IT!!!

Resources

Attachment Parenting
www.attachmentparenting.org

Birth

Active Birth Centre
London, UK
Tel: 020 7281 6760
www.activebirthcentre.com

Bumi Sehat Foundation International (Birth/Health Centre)
Founder: Robin Lim
Bali, Indonesia
www.bumisehatbali.org

Birth Crisis
www.birthcrisis.sheilakitzinger.org

Childbirth.org
www.childbirth.org

International Childbirth Education Association (ICEA)
Minneapolis, USA
www.icea.org

Lamaze Institute for Normal Birth
Washington, USA
www.lamaze.org/institute

Maternity Coalition Australia
www.maternity.coalition.org.au

National Childbirth Trust (NCT)
www.nctpregnancyandbabycare.com

Trauma and Birth Stress (TABS)
www.tabs.org.nz

Breastfeeding Support

The Breastfeeding Network
www.breastfeedingnetwork.org.uk

La Leche League UK
www.laleche.org.uk
www.laleche.com

Caesarean

International Caesarean Awareness Network (ICAN)
www.ican-online.org

Vaginal Birth after a Caesarean (VBAC)
www.vbac.com

Creating a Positive Caesarean
http://www.birthrites.org/caesarean.html
http://www.birthcut.com/thepositivecesarean.htm

Counselling

Birth Trauma Association
Ipswich, UK
www.birthtraumaassociation.org

British Association for Counselling and Psychotherapy
www.counselling.co.uk

British Association for Sexual and Relationship Therapy
www.basrt.org.uk

Relate
Relate offers advice, relationship counselling, sex therapy, workshops, mediation, consultations and support face-to-face, by phone and through this website.
www.relate.org.uk

The Art of Birth
Offering emotional support for conception, pregnancy, birth and beyond.
Founder: Alexandra Florschutz, MA
Forest Row, UK
alex@theartofbirth.co.uk
www.theartofbirth.co.uk

Doulas

Doula UK
www.doula.org.uk

Doulas of North America (DONA)
www.dona.org

Home Birth
Home Birth Reference Site
www.homebirth.org.uk

Home Midwifery Association
www.homebirth.org.au

Maternity Services

Association for Improvements in the Maternity Services (AIMS)
www.aims.org.uk

Association of Radical Midwives
www.radmid.demon.co.uk

Birth Choice UK
www.birthchoiceuk.com

Independent Midwives Association
www.independentmidwives.org.uk

Royal College of Midwives
www.rcmnormalbirth.net

Parenting Magazines

Juno Magazine
A Natural Approach to Family Life
Founders: Emma Hiwaizi and Patricia Patterson-Vanegas
www.junomagazine.com

Mothering – The Home for Natural Family Living
www.mothering.com

The Mother Magazine
One of the first conscious parenting magazines in the UK
Founder: Veronika Robinson
www.themothermagazine.co.uk

Parenting

Steve Biddulph
Parenting expert and author of Raising Boys, Raising Girls, Secret of Happy Children, The New Manhood
www.stevebiddulph.com

Naomi Aldort
Authentic Parenting Site and author of Raising Our Children, Raising Ourselves
She offers a brilliant philosophy on Self Directed Learning (a.k.a. home education)
www.aldort.com

Pregnancy Loss
AMEND (Aiding Mothers & Fathers Experiencing Neonatal Death)
USA
www.amendinc.com

CLIMB (Centre for Loss in Multiple Birth)
USA
www.climb-support.org

The Compassionate Friends
USA www.compassionatefriends.org
Canada www.tcfcanada.net
UK www.tcf.org.uk

Hygeia
USA
www.hygeia.org

Miscarriage Association
UK
www.miscarriageassociation.org.uk

Perinatal Bereavement Services of Ontario
Canada
www.pbso.ca

Pregnancy Loss Support Program
USA
www.ncjwny.org/services_plsp.htm

RESOLVE (National Fertility Association)
USA
www.resolve.org

SANDS (Stillbirth and Neonatal Death Support) UK www.uk-sands.org
AUSTRALIA www.sands.org.au
INCIID (International Council on Infertility Information Dissemination)
USA www.inciid.org

Research

Dr Michel Odent – Primal Health Research
Dr Michel Odent is a retired doctor and obstetrician, known for his role in the natural childbirth movement and for promoting water birth.
www.birthworks.org/primalhealth
www.michelodent.com

Resources Continued

Babies Know
Creating a great relationship with your kids.
www.babiesknow.com

Barry Durdant-Hollamby
Intuitive Coach/Counsellor
Email: artofchange@msn.com
www.barrydurdant-hollamby.com,

Binnie A. Dansby
Inspiring educator, therapist, philosopher and author for almost thirty years. In 1988 she created the SOURCE Process and Breathwork therapy training manual which is a specifically designed system for personal and professional development. The purpose of this system is to facilitate the safe and effective release and healing of the life-long wounds of fear, inadequacy and limitation. It is designed to empower each person through the use of practical and powerful tools, techniques, inspiration, and the breath.

Her Empowering Birth Program of birth preparation has been of great support to women in many countries. She and Lynne Thorsen Rowe are currently writing the Wake up Series about creating Ecstatic Birth and Ecstatic Life.
www.binnieadansby.com

Birthing From Within
www.birthingfromwithin.com

Birthlight Trust
Offers simple body-based practices inspired from yoga and traditional modes of parenting.
Aims to enhance the health and wellbeing of women and their families from conception through to the third year.
www.birthlight.com

Fathers To Be
A superb resource addressing the needs of fathers in the transition to fatherhood.
Founder: Patrick Houser
www.fatherstobe.org

Foresight
Preconception Support
www.foresight-preconception.org.uk

The International Professional Breathwork Alliance
A consortium of professional schools, trainers and practitioners who support and promote the integration of Breathwork in the world as an accessible and vital healing modality that facilitates physical, emotional and spiritual wellness.
www.breathworkalliance.com

International Breathwork Foundation
Organisation for international Breathworkers.
www.ibfnetwork.org

Kundalini Yoga
www.devotion.org.uk

Mother's Milk Books
Editor: Teika Bellamy
UK
teika@mothersmilkbooks.com
www.mothersmilkbooks.com

"The ambition of Mother's Milk Books is to publish books for children and adults that normalise breastfeeding. There are very few books on the market that illustrate the natural beauty of the breastfeeding mother-baby dyad, and we at Mother's Milk Books would like to change that! To find out more about our forthcoming projects, and to buy our first title Musings on Mothering, an anthology of art, poetry, and prose, please visit our website."

Pat Bennaceur (BACP)
Psychotherapist, SOURCE Breathwork Therapist.
Email: patbennaceur@freenetname.co.uk
www.re-birth.uk.com

Sacred Birthing
A Spiritual Perspective on Childbirth
www.sacredbirthing.com

The Secret Club Project
Founder: Laura Seftel
UK
www.secretclubproject.org

Water Birth Website
www.waterbirthinfo.com

Bibliography

Aldort, N. (2009) *Raising Our Children, Raising Ourselves*. USA: Book Publishers Network.

Balaskas, J. (2004) *The Water Birth Book*. London: Thorsons.

Barber, V. (2002) *Explore yourself through Art*. London: Carroll & Brown Ltd

Baring, A., & Cashford, J. (1991) *The Myth of the Goddess: Evolution of an Image*. London: Penguin Books Ltd.

Bergum, V. (1989) *Woman to Mother: A Transformation*. London: Granby, Mass: Bergin & Garvey Publishers.

Biddulph, Steve & Sharon (2000) *Love, Laughter & Parenting – in the precious years from birth to six*. London: Dorling Kindersley Ltd.

Bion, W. R. (1991) *Experiences in Groups – and other papers*. London, USA, Canada: Routledge.

Bowlby, J. (2005) *A Secure Base*. London, NY, Canada: Routledge.

Case, C. and Dalley, T. (2002) *The Handbook of Art Therapy*. Hove, NY: Brunner-Routledge.

Cameron, J. (1997) *The Vein of Gold – A Journey to your Creative Heart*. London: Pan Books.

Camphausen, R. C. (1996) *The Yoni – Sacred Symbol of Female Creative Power*. Rochester, Vermont: Inner Traditions International.

Case, C., & Dalley, T. (2002) *The Handbook of Art Therapy*. Hove: Brunner-Routledge.

Chamberlain, D. B. (1998) *The Mind of Your Newborn Baby*. USA: North Atlantic Books.

Coleman, A. M. (2003) *Oxford Dictionary of Psychology*. UK: Oxford University Press.

Cotterell, A., & Storm, R. (1999) *The Ultimate Encyclopedia of Mythology*. UK: Hermes House.

Dansby, B. A. (1996) *Birth of a Rebirther*. Sweden: Archie Duncanson. (1998) *Healing Birth – The Transformation of Life*. Germany: Midwives Congress, May 1998.

Dick-Read, G. (2006) *Childbirth without Fear*. London: Pollinger in Print.

Drake, S. (1979) *The Path to Birth*. Edinburgh: Floris Books.

Edwards, D. (2004) *Art Therapy*. London: Sage Publications Ltd.

Furin, K. (2005) *Healing Sexual Abuse through Natural Childbirth*. The Mother Magazine. Cumbria UK: Veronika Sophia Robinson.

Furth, G. M. (2002) *The Secret World of Drawings: A Jungian Approach to Healing Through Art*. Canada: Inner City Books.

Eiseman, JR. B. (1990) *Bali: Sekala and Niskala*. Asia, Australia, Indonesia, Japan, UK and USA. Periplus Editions.

England, P., Horowitz, R. (1998) *Birthing from within – an Extra-Ordinary Guide to Childbirth Preparation*. New Mexico: Partera Press.

Estes, C. P. (1998) *Women Who Run With The Wolves*. London: Rider. (2012) *Seeing in the Dark – Myths & Stories to Reclaim the Buried, Knowing Woman*. USA: Sounds True. CD.

Gaskin, I. M. (2002) *Spiritual Midwifery*. USA: Book Publishing Company.

Gelder, N., Mayor, R., Cowen, P. (2001) *Shortter Oxford Text Book of Psychiatry*. Oxford: Oxford University Press (p497-503).

Gerhardt, S. (2004) *Why Love Matters*. East Sussex & New York: Brunner-Routledge.

Hay, L. (2007) *You Can Heal Your Life*. Australia, Canada, Hong Kong, India-South Africa, UK and USA: Hay House, Inc.

Hogan, S. (ed) (1997) *Feminist Approaches to Art Therapy*. London, New York: Routledge.

Horovitz-Darby, E. G. (1994) *Spiritual Art Therapy: An Alternate Path*. USA: Charles C Thomas Publisher

Houser, P. M. (2007) *Fathers-To-Be Handbook – A Roadmap for the Transition to Fatherhood*. UK: Creative Life Systems UK.

Holmes, J. (1999) *John Bowlby & Attachment Theory*. London & USA: Routledge.

Jung, C. G. (1986) *Four Archetypes: Mother, Rebirth, Spirit, Trickster*. (Eds) Read, H. (d. 1968), Fordham, M., & Adler, G. London: Ark Paperbacks.
(1978) *Man and His Symbols*. London: Pan Books.
(1992) *Jung for Beginners*. (Eds) Hyde, M., & McGuinness, M. Cambridge: Icon Books Ltd.

Killick, K. and Schaverien, J. (eds) (1997) *Art Psychotherapy and Psychosis*. London, NY: Routledge.

Kitzinger, S. (2007) *Birth Crisis*. London: Routledge.

Larousse Encyclopaedia of Mythology (1959) London: Batchworth Press Ltd.

Leboyer, F. (1991) *Birth without Violence*. London: Mandarin Paperbacks.

Leeming, D., & Page, J. (1994) *Myths of the Female Divine Goddess*. Oxford, USA: Oxford University Press.

Liebmann, M. (1986) *Art Therapy for Groups – a handbook of Themes, Games and Exercises*. Newton MA: Brookline Books.

Liedloff, J. (2004) *The Continuum Concept*. London: Penguin Books.

Lievegoed, B. (1993) *Phases: The Spiritual Rhythms of Adult Life*. Bristol: Rudolf Steiner Press.
(1997) *Phases of Childhood: Growing in Body, Soul & Spirit*. Edinburgh: Floris Books.

Lipton, B., H. (2009) *Biology of Belief*. USA: Hay House, Inc.

Lord, A. (2010) *Colour Dynamics – Workbook for Watercolour Painting and Colour Theory*. Gloucestershire UK: Hawthorn Press.

Malchiodi, C. A. (1998) *The Art Therapy Sourcebook*. Los Angeles: Lowell House.

McNeilly, G. (2006) *Group Analytic Art Therapy*. London, USA: Jessica Kingsley Publishers.

Miller, A. (2006) *The Body Never Lies – The Lingering Effects of Hurtful Parenting.* London, New York: W. W. Norton & Company. (1995) *The Drama of Being a Child.* London: Virago.

Miller, L., Rustin, M., Rustin, M., Shuttleworth, J. (Edited By) (1991) *Closely Observed Infants.* London: Gerald Duckworth & Co. Ltd.

Northrup, C. (2009) *Women's Bodies, Women's Wisdom – The Complete Guide to Women's Health and Wellbeing.* UK: Piatkus.

Odent, M. (1999) *The Scientification of Love.* London: Free Association Books.

Piontelli, A. (1997) *From Foetus to Child: An Observational & Psychoanalytic study.* London, USA & Canada: Routledge.

Rank, O. (1968) *Art & Artist.* New York: Agathon Press, Inc.

Raphael-Leff, J. (1995) *Pregnancy: The Inside Story.* London & New Jersey: Jason Aronson Inc.

Scott, Y., Jenkins, R. (1998) *Psychiatric Disorders Specific to Women in: Companion to Psychiatric Studies 6th Ed.* Churchill Livingston. (p556).

Schaverien, J. (1999) *The Revealing Image.* London, USA: Jessica Kingsley Publishers.

Shinoda Bolen, J. (1984) *Goddesses in Every Woman.* New York: Harper & Row, Publishers, Inc.

Skaife, S. and Huet, V. (eds) (1998) *Art Psychotherapy Groups – Between Pictures and Words.* London, USA, Canada: Routledge

St-Andre, M. (1993) *Psychotherapy during Pregnancy: Opportunities & Challenges* American Journal of Psychotherapy, Vol. 47, No. 4 Autumn.

Stern, D. N. (2004) *The Interpersonal World of the Infant: A View from Psychoanalysis & Developmental Psychology.* London: Karnac (Books) Ltd.

Steiner, R. (Translated by John Salter & Pauline Wehrle) (2005) Colour (12 Lectures). Forest Row, UK: Rudolph Steiner Press. (2003) *Isis, Mary, Sophia – Her Mission and Ours.* USA: Steiner Books. (1968) *The Fifth Gospel.* London: Rudolph Steiner Press.

Stewart, W. (1996) *Imagery & Symbolism in Counselling.* London & USA: Jessica Kingsley Publishers Ltd.
(1998) *Dictionary of Imagery & Symbolism in Counselling.* London: Jessica Kingsley Publishers Ltd.

Swan-Foster, N. (1989) *Images of Pregnant Women: Art Therapy as a Tool for Transformation.* USA: The Arts in Psychotherapy, Vol 16, pp. 283-292.

Swinglehurst, E. (1995) *The Art of the Surrealists.* New York: Shooting Star Press.

Symington, J. (1996) *The Clinical Thinking of Wilfred Bion.* London: Routledge.

Szasz, T. S. (1974) *The Myth of Mental Illness.* New York: Harper & Row Publishers.

Taylor, C. L. (1991) *The Inner Child Workbook.* New York: Tarcher/Penguin.

Thomas, Glyn V. & Silk, Angele M. J. (1989) *An Introduction to the Psychology of Children's Drawings.* London: Harvester Wheatsheaf.

Thomashauer, R. (2003) *Mama Gena's School of Womanly Arts.* New York: Simon & Schuster.

Verny, T. (1981) *The Secret Life of the Unborn Child.* New York: Dell Publishing.

Virtue, D. (2004) *Angel Medicine – How to heal the body and mind with the help of the angels.* London: Hay House UK Ltd and worldwide.

Waller, D. (2004) *Group Interactive Art Therapy.* Hove, NY: Brunner-Routledge.

Weihs, T. (1986) *Embryogenesis in Myth & Science.* Edinburgh: Floris Books.

Winnicott, D. W. (1971) *Playing & Reality.* London: Tavistock Publications.

Wolf, N. (2002) *Misconceptions – Truth, Lies and the Unexpected on the Journey to Motherhood.* London: Vintage (Random House).
(2012) *Vagina – A New Biography.* London: Virago.

Yalom, I. D. (1983) *Inpatient Group Psychotherapy.* USA: Basic Books.

Films:

Birth Reborn by Michel Odent 1992, BBC Documentary Video.

Life before Birth. Channel 4 Documentary April 2005. Written, Directed, & Produced by Toby Macdonald. Pioneer Productions.

Observation Observed – Closely Observed Infants on Film. The Tavistock Clinic Foundation Film using observational material from the BBC. Written by Margaret Rustin and Beth Miller.

Orgasmic Birth – the best kept secret. Directed by Debra Pascali-Bonaro & Produced by Debra Pascali-Bonaro & Kris Liem. 2008 Sunken Treasuer, LLC.

The Psychology of Birth: Invitation to Intimacy. Directed/Produced by Elmer Postle. Narrated by Binnie A. Dansby.

The Business of being Born. Documentary Film produced by Ricki Lake 2008. This film explores the contemporary experience of childbirth in the United States.
http://www.thebusinessofbeingborn.com/

Research Web Sites:

www.birthworks.org/primalhealth
www.birthalliance.com
www.birth.net
www.birthinternational.co.uk
www.birthpsychology.com (APPPAH)
www.childbirth.org
www.e-pregnancy.com

www.pregnancy.org
www.themothermagazine.co.uk

Papers found on www.birthinternational.com

Chamberlain, D., Ph.D., - *Introduction to Life Before Birth*
                              - Prenatal Memory and Learning

Haire, D., (1994) *Obstetric Drugs & Procedures: their Effects on Mother & Baby*, Paper presented at the Future Birth Conference, Australia. My reference was cited in *The Pain of Labour – A Feminist Issue* by Andrea Robertson

Robertson, A., - *Are Midwives a Dying Breed?* The Practicing Midwife, Vol. 5, No. 7. (2002)
                        - The Pain of Labour – A Feminist Issue
                        - Working with the Young and Pregnant
                        - The Power of the Group
                        - Watch Your Language
                        - Help – it hurts – get me the Complementary Therapies!
                        - Get the Fathers Involved

These articles were found on www.birthinternational.com but were probably published in The Practicing Midwife as well. Dates and references were not given.

Changesurfer Consulting. The Medical Literature on The Safety of Home Birth www.changesurfer.com/Hlth/homebirth/html

International Society of Prenatal & Perinatal Psychology & Medicine (ISPPM) www.isppm.com

National Birthday Trust – Report of the Confidential Enquiry into Home Births. Home Birth Reference Site. www.homebirth.org.uk/homebirth2.html

National Institute for Mental Health in England (NIMHE) (2005) Women's Birth Experience. www.nimhe.csip.org.uk

British Medical Journal (2005; 230:1416, 18 June) Outcomes of Planned Home Births with Certified Midwives: Large Prospective Study in North America. www.bmj.bmjjournals.com

Inscape Journal of Art Therapy

NCBI (A service of the National Library of Medicine and the National Institutes of Health). Articles on home birth/hospital birth. www.ncbi.nlm.nih.gov www.pubmed.gov

TNS System Three (prepared by) (October 2005), NHS Maternity Services Quantitative Research. TNS System Three, Edinburgh.

Research on Maternity Services, Statistics, Costs, etc:
Department of Health on Maternity Services

Kings Fund

House of Commons Health Committee – Provision of Maternity Services 2002/03

ISPPM

The Information Centre (NHS)

HOSPITAL EPISODE STATISTICS: NHS Maternity Statistics, 2010-11 (HES online Office for national statistics – Home births 2010

The Sainsbury Centre for Mental Health: www.scmh.org.uk

1. Briefing 16: An Executive Briefing on adult acute in-patient care for people with mental health problems.

The Royal College of Psychiatrists: www.rcpsych.ac.uk
https://catalogue.ic.nhs.uk/publications/hospital/maternity/nhs-mater-eng-2011-2012/nhs-mate-eng-2011-2012-rep.pdf

Lightning Source UK Ltd.
Milton Keynes UK
UKOW06f0726161013

219146UK00003B/5/P